Rapamycin, mTOR, Autophagy & Treating mTOR Syndrome

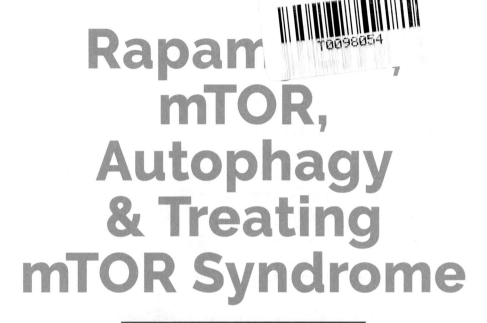

RAPAMYCIN
The Most Promising
Life Extension Drug

By Ross Pelton, *The Natural Pharmacist*

Updated 2nd edition

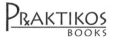

PRAKTIKOS
BOOKS

What the Experts Are Saying

"Ross Pelton's new book, *Rapamycin, mTOR, Autophagy & Treating mTOR Syndrome,* is a timely introduction to this exciting area of longevity research. Based on solid science, and written in an accurate and accessible manner, this book provides readers with foundational knowledge to begin their own journey toward optimal healthspan."

— **Matt Kaeberlein, PhD, Professor of Laboratory Medicine and Pathology, University of Washington**

"Ross Pelton has done a remarkable job making a very complex subject understandable in clear and simple language. It provides a very good balance between references to studies without getting lost in the details. Rapamycin is one of the great new drugs of the past 100 years. This is a very good and very courageous effort to introduce rapamycin to the general public. This is a very important book that everybody should read. [In fact,] reading this book might add years to your life."

— **Alan Green, MD**

"Ross Pelton's book, *Rapamycin, mTOR, Autophagy & Treating mTOR Syndrome*, explains how rapamycin has the promise of increasing the lifespan and, more importantly, the healthspan of individuals by increasing autophagy and slowing the aging process. This book will reveal an additional way for you to get onto a path of health and wellness, naturally."

— **Steven F. Hotze, MD, CEO, Hotze Health & Wellness Center, Houston, TX**

"Do not allow the title *Rapamycin, mTOR, Autophagy & Treating mTOR Syndrome* to deter you from reading Ross Pelton's most recent book ASAP! If you desire to stay as healthy as possible for as long possible, ***Rapamycin*** should be on your must-read list. Dr. Pelton helps bring to bear an expeditious way to slow down the process of aging, but without the hardship and punitive experience of fasting."

**— Dr. Bob Martin, host of the *Dr. Bob Martin Show*,
the largest syndicated radio health talk show in the U.S.**

"*Rapamycin, mTOR, Autophagy & Treating mTOR Syndrome* is a beautifully balanced book which lays out the case for rapamycin with scholarly rigor that's easily accessible and actionable. Count on Ross Pelton to always be on the cutting edge!"

**— Dr. Ron Hoffman, host of Intelligent Medicine,
the longest-running MD-hosted health show
on syndicated radio**

"Is rapamycin the long-sought fountain of youth? Ross Pelton's short, easy-to-read book on rapamycin and its anti-aging effects on animals makes one ask why are there so few human studies and why physicians are largely unfamiliar with it. The fact that rapamycin is produced by a strain of bacteria found in the soil on Easter Island only makes its potential use even more compelling. Pelton explains why rapamycin, which may be a lifesaving drug for organ trans-plant patients, is also an effective life extension drug."

— Jonathan Collin, MD, Publisher, *Townsend Letter*

Praktikos Books
94 Landfill Road
Edinburg, VA 22824
888-542-9467

Rapamycin, mTOR, Autophagy & Treating mTOR Syndrome 2nd edition © 2023 by Ross Pelton. All rights reserved. Printed in the United States of America. No part of this book may be used or reproduced in any manner whatsoever without written permission except in the case of brief quotations used in critical articles and reviews.

www.naturalpharmacist.net

Praktikos books are produced in alliance with Axios Press.

Library of Congress Cataloging-in-Publication Data

Names: Pelton, Ross, author.
Title: Rapamycin, mTOR, autophagy & treating mTOR syndrome : rapamycin, the
   most promising life extension drug / by Ross Pelton, the Natural
   Pharmacist.
Other titles: Rapamycin, mTOR, autophagy and treating mTOR syndrome
Description: Updated 2nd edition. | Edinburg, VA : Praktikos Books, [2023]
   | Revised edition of: Rapamycin, mTOR, autophagy & treating mTOR
   syndrome / by Ross Pelton, the Natural Pharmacist. [2022]. | Includes
   bibliographical references and index. | Summary: "Rapamycin is the most
   promising life extension drug ever discovered. mTOR and autophagy are a
   breakthrough in our understanding of aging. Rapamycin helps re-balance
   the mTOR/autophagy ratio to delay the onset of age-related diseases.
   Rapamycin, mTOR, Autophagy & Treating mTOR Syndrome is a book about how
   to successfully increase health-span and lifespan. This book includes
   updated information"-- Provided by publisher.
Identifiers: LCCN 2023014084 (print) | LCCN 2023014085 (ebook) | ISBN
   9781607660170 (paperback) | ISBN 9781607660187 (ebook)
Subjects: LCSH: Rapamycin.
Classification: LCC RM373 .P45 2023 (print) | LCC RM373 (ebook) | DDC
   615.3/7--dc23/eng/20230414
LC record available at https://lccn.loc.gov/2023014084
LC ebook record available at https://lccn.loc.gov/2023014085

To my loving wife, Taffy

You enrich my life beyond my ability to express
my appreciation and thanks to you.

Thanks for understanding my passion and my need
to write and communicate about health to the world.

Thanks for continually bringing love, laughter,
and spontaneity into my life.

Thanks for your patience, your understanding, your wisdom,
and....thanks for being my wife and my best friend!

Hello, Readers,

The information in this book is a paradigm shift, a breakthrough, and a revolutionary new understanding of cellular biochemistry, health and the aging process.

mTOR and autophagy are scientific/medical discoveries of historic proportions. These cellular mechanisms regulate the health and the aging process of every living organism, especially humans. The purpose of this book is to explain mTOR and autophagy, the counterbalancing relationship between them, and how rapamycin can help correct an imbalance in the mTOR/autophagy ratio.

The information in this book can help improve peoples' health, delay the onset of age-related diseases, and extend the lifespan and healthspan of most people alive today.

Please share this book with others.

Let's make good health go viral!

Thanks, Ross

TABLE OF CONTENTS

PREFACE

> 66 From extending lifespan to bolstering the immune system, rapamycin's effects are only just beginning to be understood. 99
>
> *The Scientist: March 1, 2018*

There are two themes that are central to this book:

Theme #1 is the story of rapamycin, perhaps the most promising life-extension drug that has ever been discovered.

Rapamycin is the common name for the Pfizer-owned drug named Rapamune, which has a generic name **sirolimus**.

Theme #2 is story of mTOR and autophagy, which grew out of the research conducted to understand rapamycin's mechanism of action. Learning about mTOR and autophagy has resulted in the discovery of a fundamental process within all cells that regulates health and the aging process.

There are fundamental new *Rules of Health* for people to learn in order to lead a healthy life. Unfortunately, when it comes to health, most people, including myself, have not had good teachers and role models. The rapamycin story, which includes mTOR and autophagy, explains a fundamental biochemical mechanism that regulates the health and lifespan of every cell in your body; it is one of the most important *Rules of Health* for people to understand.

mTOR Syndrome

I've coined a new term: *mTOR Syndrome,* which results from the overexpression of a cellular enzyme called **mTOR** coupled with the under-activity of a cell housekeeping process called **autophagy**. mTOR and autophagy will be thoroughly explained in this book. Rapamycin is the most effective drug yet discovered to treat mTOR Syndrome.

mTOR Syndrome is a major contributing factor to the epidemic of chronic degenerative diseases; it helps explain why sub-optimal health is so widespread and discusses important options people can take to help improve the quality and quantity of their life.

The rapamycin story is fairly new. Until now, only the scientists who have conducted studies and a few life extension enthusiasts are familiar with these topics. But this information is just beginning to reach the public.

The goal of my book is to help change this by explaining why and how rapamycin (and several other therapies) can help you improve your health and "move your needle" in the direction of improved health and slowing down your biological aging process…i.e. healthy life extension, or healthy longevity.

As important and effective as rapamycin is, it is not a miracle drug that is going to make everyone who takes it return to good health. There are many factors that contribute to poor health, just as there are many lifestyle components that promote good health.

My point is this: overall, rapamycin is a very important, very effective drug that holds the potential to improve the health and lives of untold millions of people now living. However, it is my opinion that integrating additional health-promoting modalities into your life along with rapamycin will increase and accelerate improvements in your health.

On the other hand, I also believe that a smoker who drinks alcohol, eats junk food and doesn't exercise is not likely to get much benefit from taking rapamycin. A multitude of bad habits and choices will likely override rapamycin's potential benefits.

My goals for writing this book are the following:

a. I want to provide readers with a summary of the history, development, and benefits of rapamycin so that you understand its potential benefit for you and your loved ones.

b. I want to "coach" readers on how to use this information to educate your physician about rapamycin and give you pointers on how to ask your physician to prescribe rapamycin for you. Let's face it, in the U.S., physicians must write a prescription for rapamycin. Therefore, educating physicians about rapamycin is critical in order to increase awareness and use of rapamycin.

c. To facilitate and accelerate everyone's rapamycin/mTOR/autophagy learning curve, I have provided links in Chapter 10 to key scientific studies, articles, and podcast interviews on rapamycin.

d. I will discuss dosages, directions, side effects (it is quite safe) and how to find a pharmacy that will fill your prescription for rapamycin.

I urge you to educate yourself about rapamycin, educate your physician about rapamycin and help me educate the world about the amazing health benefits of rapamycin.

Here's to increasing your healthy longevity.

In gratitude,

Ross Pelton, Ph.D.

The Natural Pharmacist

INTRODUCTION

This book will explain how the following three terms provide a new understanding of the mechanisms that regulate health and the aging process in all living organisms, from single cell organisms up to and including humans. These three terms are:

» rapamycin

» mTOR

» and autophagy

mTOR and autophagy have been regulating the health of all life forms since life began to emerge on Earth in single cell organisms approximately 3.5 billion years ago.

After the discovery of rapamycin, scientists began conducting experiments in an effort to understand rapamycin's mechanism of action. This led to the discovery of mTOR, which in turn, led to the understanding of how mTOR and autophagy regulate cellular metabolism and ultimately, the health and life of all living things.

In summary, the discovery of rapamycin resulted in scientific studies that have enabled scientists to gain a totally new understanding of the aging process and how we might use this new information to improve health and delay the onset of age-related diseases. Collectively, the topics in this book describe one of the most important breakthroughs in the science of life extension that have ever been discovered.

Rapamycin works by shifting the body's cellular biochemistry into a mode that mimics calorie restriction. This sets a cascade of beneficial effects in motion at the cellular level, which improves health, delays the onset of many diseases, and increases lifespan.

Rapamycin treatment has increased lifespan from 25–60% in most species it has been tested on. When rapamycin was given to 20-month (elderly) mice, females lived 14% longer and males lived 9% longer.[1] These results suggest that rapamycin started late in life may also improve health and extend lifespan in humans.

The following image shows the exciting potential of synergistic effects of combining rapamycin with other health-promoting substances. The study in the box shows that combining rapamycin with lithium and a senolytic drug extended fruit fly lifespans by 48%. Even a 10%–15% increase in fruit fly lifespan is considered remarkable.

Lithium is a low-cost dietary supplement that can safely be taken in the dose of 1000 mcg a day without the side effects caused by far higher prescription drug doses.

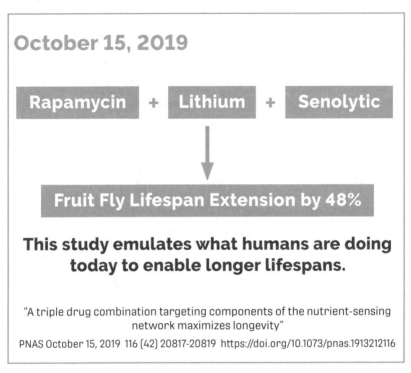

In 1935, a landmark study was published, which reported that laboratory rats placed on a calorie restricted diet, while maintaining adequate nutrition, lived 33% longer than previously known possible.[2] Since that time, many experiments on a wide range of animals have confirmed that calorie restricted diets, without malnutrition, can achieve significant increases in lifespan. Rapamycin mimics calorie restriction.[3,4]

Discovery of Rapamycin

Rapamycin is a compound that is produced by a strain of bacteria named *Streptomyces rapamycinicus* (previously classified as *Streptomyces hygroscopicus*). This bacterium was discovered from soil samples taken during a scientific expedition to Easter Island in 1964. The purpose of this scientific expedition was to search for compounds that might express antifungal and/or antibiotic properties.

Although rapamycin exhibited strong anti-fungal activity, efforts to market it as an antifungal drug were discontinued when it was discovered to have potent immunosuppressive activity when taken in daily doses. Subsequently, rapamycin was approved by the FDA in September 1999 as a drug to prevent organ transplant rejection.

Additional studies revealed that rapamycin exhibits a broad range of other functions. Promising results from initial studies prompted scientists to send samples of rapamycin to the U.S. National Cancer Institute (NCI) for further testing.

Initial tests at the National Cancer Institute revealed that rapamycin had activity against solid tumors. Subsequently, the NCI elevated rapamycin to *priority drug* status because of its anti-cancer activity and because it functioned differently than most anticancer drugs.[5]

Many anticancer drugs are classified as "cytotoxic drugs" because they kill rapidly dividing cancer cells. However, cytotoxicity causes a wide range of side effects because other rapidly dividing cells such as bone marrow cells and cells lining the intestinal tract also sustain significant damage. Rapamycin appeared to be a totally new type of anticancer drug because it functioned by inhibiting cancer growth (cytostatic) rather than by killing cancer cells (cytotoxic).

LIFE EXTENSION: The most exciting news about rapamycin is in the field of life extension. Rapamycin has produced important health improvements and/or significant life extension in every species tested thus far, which includes yeast, worms, fruit flies[6] and mice. The results of these studies suggest that rapamycin is the most effective life extension drug ever discovered.

An important factor in rapamycin's favor is the fact that scientists now understand how and why rapamycin produces so many beneficial effects. Rapamycin functions by entering cells and binding to an enzyme named mTOR. mTOR is a fundamental mechanism within all cells that regulates the production of proteins, enzymes, and processes of cellular growth and metabolism.

Current life extension clinical trials are underway with dogs, marmosets (a tiny monkey that only lives to about eight years old), and humans. Regarding testing rapamycin in humans, in June of 2021, a crowdfunding project successfully raised $485,000 for the first human rapamycin clinical trial. This is called the PEARL trial, which stands for *The Participatory Evaluation (of) Aging (with) Rapamycin (for) Longevity Study.*[7]

The box below provides a brief summary of this study and a log in web address on how you can enroll:

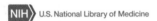 U.S. National Library of Medicine

ClinicalTrials.gov   June 18, 2021

Rapamycin Human Study Receives $485,000 Funding

» Randomized, placebo-controlled trial into the safety/efficacy of rapamycin in reducing clinical measures of aging in an older adult population.

» The differing doses: 5 mg or 10 mg of rapamycin one time a week or placebo.

» Primary Outcome Measure: Changes in visceral fat as measured by (DXA) scan.

» Secondary Outcomes: Range of clinical measures, e.g. bone density, blood tests, etc.

» 20 people enrolled at $360 each (original cost before donations was $1,200).

Principal investigators: **James Watson, M.D.** and **Sajad Zalzala, M.D.**

Sponsor: **AgelessRx**

Collaborator: **University of California, Los Angeles**

To enroll log on to: **https://www.agelessrx.com/pearl**

CHAPTER ONE

Key Bullet Points Summarizing Rapamycin

- Rapamycin is a potent antifungal/antibiotic drug that was discovered in 1964 in a soil sample taken from Easter Island; the first study on rapamycin was published in 1975 (as an antifungal agent).

- Rapamycin was approved by the FDA in September 1999 as a drug to prevent organ transplant rejection.

- Mechanism of action:

  a. Inhibits the signaling pathway named mTOR (explained in Part 4).

  b. Mimics calorie restriction.

  c. Activates autophagy: the body's mechanism for cellular repair, regeneration, and detoxification.

- Rapamycin has been used safely in humans for decades; it is FDA approved for prevention of organ transplant rejection, as a treatment for certain types of cancer, and in patients receiving cardiac stents.

- In one of the first life extension studies, rapamycin given to 20-month-old (elderly) mice increased median lifespan of females 14% and males 9%.[8] In a subsequent trial with 9-month-old (young) mice given 3x greater dose of rapamycin, median lifespan increased 26% in females and 23% in males.[9]

- In 2006, Dr. Mikhail Blagosklonny was the first to propose that **"rapamycin could be used immediately to slow down aging and all age-related diseases in humans, thus becoming an anti-aging drug today."**[10,11]

- Rapamycin is administered every day to inhibit rejection in organ transplant patients; when it is given at lower doses (once weekly) rapamycin improves many health metrics and is associated with life extension.

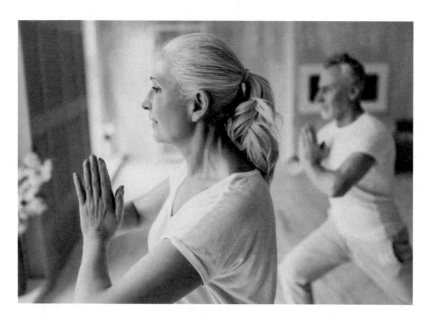

- Rapamycin has produced significant life extension in every species tested including yeast, worms, fruit flies, and mice. Currently clinical trials are also being conducted in dogs and marmosets (a tiny primate/monkey that only lives to about eight years old).

- Joan Mannick, M.D. conducted the first clinical trial which revealed that low-dose rapamycin-like drugs strengthen the immune system in elderly humans.[12]

> ❝ From 2009 through 2016, approximately 180 papers/year have been published on rapamycin and aging. ❞

- The first ever human rapamycin life extension trial (PEARL trial) has been funded and will begin soon. PEARL stands for the *Participatory Evaluation (of) Aging (with) Rapamycin (for) Longevity Study*. This study was funded in a crowdfunding campaign that raised $485,000.

- There has been an explosion of rapamycin research. From the first published rapamycin study in 1975 until 2008, there were fewer than 10 published papers per year on the topic of "rapamycin and aging." However, from 2009 through 2016,

approximately 180 papers/year have been published on rapamycin and aging. A PubMed search
on January 6, 2022, showed 6,358 listings with the
word rapamycin in the title.

Key Benefits of Taking Rapamycin

Taking rapamycin helps all cells in the body begin
to function better; it slows the process of aging.
Improvements are reported in a wide range of
chronic degenerative diseases.

The most commonly reported benefits, which have
mostly been documented in animal models, include
the following:

a. Weight loss (significantly in the abdominal region)[13]

b. Improvements in hearing, eyesight and cognitive
function

c. Gains in energy, strength, stamina, and endurance

d. Delaying the onset of many age-related diseases
including cancers, neurological diseases, and
diabetes

e. Enhances certain immune functions

f. Reduces the incidence of age-related diseases,
including cancer, cognitive decline, neurodegeneration, cardiovascular disease, and diabetes

CHAPTER TWO

History and Discovery of Rapamycin

The fascinating story of the discovery of rapamycin and the mTOR signaling pathway began in 1964 when a team of Canadian scientists embarked on scientific expedition to Easter Island to search for new antimicrobial agents. A microbiologist named Georges Nogrady, who was employed by the drug company Ayerst Pharmaceuticals, brought some soil samples from Easter Island back to his lab in Montreal.

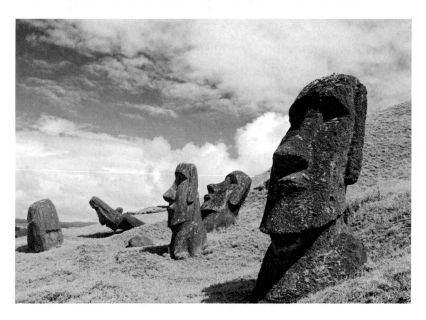

EASTER ISLAND (RAPA NUI)

Easter Island is one of the most remote places on earth. It is located in the Pacific Ocean, 2,290 miles west of Chile, 2,629 miles east of Tahiti and 4,483 miles from Hawaii. Easter Island is VERY remote. So, why did a group of Canadian scientists choose Easter Island as the site for their scientific expedition in 1964? The scientists, who worked for Ayerst Pharmaceuticals, were looking for sources for new antibiotics and/or anti-fungal drugs. What they found was both unexpected and remarkable.

For centuries, horses have run wild and free on Easter Island. In fact, horses actually outnumber the island's human inhabitants. During their exploration, the Ayerst researchers noted that the tetanus bacterium is commonly found in areas where there are horses. This led the lead scientist, Georges Nogrady, to wonder why the natives on Easter Island, who constantly walked barefoot, never contracted tetanus. Nogrady returned to Canada with 67 soil samples from Easter Island. One of those soil samples contained a unique species of bacteria named *Streptomyces hygroscopicus*, which produces a compound that that Nogrady named rapamycin, after Rapa Nui, the indigenous people's name for Easter Island.

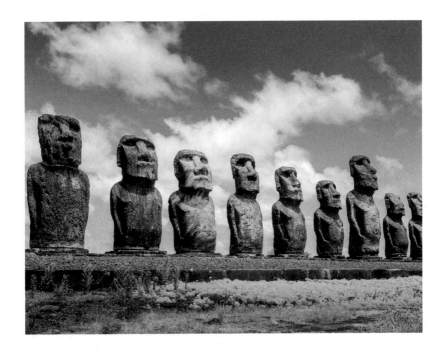

One of Dr. Nogrady's soil samples contained a strain of bacteria named *Streptomyces hygroscopicus*, which produced a compound that exhibited anti-fungal properties. After two years of study, the structure of the compound was identified and given the name rapamycin. The name rapamycin was based on Rapa Nui, which is the name the indigenous people called their island. In 1722, Dutch explorers renamed the island Easter Island. It is located about 2,300 miles from Chile's west coast and 2,500 miles east of Tahiti. Today, Easter Island is most famous for the existence of nearly 900 giant stone statues that were created by the inhabitants between the 13th and 16th centuries.

Rapamycin was initially developed as an antifungal drug. Years later, it was discovered that rapamycin was an immunosuppressant, which resulted in rapamycin being approved by the FDA as an immuno- suppressant drug to prevent organ rejection in patients who received a kidney transplant.

> NCI testing revealed that rapamycin exhibited remarkable activity against solid tumor cancers.

Scientists also discovered that rapamycin was an antipro- liferative agent. This means it can prevent cells from multi- plying, which is an important characteristic in cancer treat- ment. These observations motivated Ayerst microbiolo- gist Suren Sehgal to send a sample of rapamycin to the U.S. National Cancer Institute (NCI) for testing.

NCI testing revealed that rapamycin exhibited remark- able activity against solid tumor cancers.[14] Subsequently, the NCI assigned rapamycin to **priority drug status** to accelerate research. It was soon learned that rapamycin was the first of a totally new class of anticancer agents, a cytostatic agent rather than a cytotoxic agent.

Cytotoxic cancer drugs cause far more side effects because they kill many rapidly dividing cells in the body, not just cancer cells.[15]

In addition to the activity and benefits previously mentioned, rapamycin is being recognized as a drug that effectively improves healthspan and lifespan, which means it may soon become a bona fide life extension drug (not all studies show anti-cancer properties).

Rapamycin Activates Genes Associated with Maximum Lifespan

Vera Gorbunova, PhD, is an endowed professor of biology at the University of Rochester and a co-director of the *Rochester Aging Research Center*. Her research is focused on understanding the mechanisms of longevity and genome stability, and on the studies of exceptionally long-lived mammals.

Long-living animals, including humans, have genes in common that both negatively and positively affect lifespan. In fact, thousands of genes have now been identified in mammals that are associated with a species' maximum lifespan (MLS), either positively (Pos-MLS) or negatively (Neg-MLS).[16]

Dr. Gorbunova examined 10 prominent life extension therapies in mice and assessed how each intervention affected the genes associated with maximum lifespan.[17]   The interventions evaluated were rapamycin, 17alpha-estradiol, pituitary-specific positive transcription Factor 1 (PIT1), growth hormone, rilmenidine, ascorbyl palmitate, acarbose, calorie restriction, methionine restriction, and protandim.

RAPAMYCIN WINS! The results from Dr. Gorbunova's study revealed that rapamycin significantly reduced the activity of genes that have a negative effect on maximum lifespan. Rapamycin therapy also substantially increased the activity of genes positively associated with maximum lifespan (see image below).

mTOR Syndrome refers to the constant overexpression of mTOR, and the corresponding under-expression of autophagy. An increasing number of scientific studies suggests that this dysfunction contributes to and accelerates the onset of virtually all age-related diseases.

Rapamycin enters cells and binds to mTOR. As a result, partially inhibiting mTOR with rapamycin enables the cellular process of autophagy to be activated. Some of rapamycin's benefits may be related to its influence on the genes associated with maximum lifespan, activating genes associated with maximum lifespan and having a minimal effect on genes associated with accelerated aging.

Although Professor Gorbunova's study was not a human clinical trial, it provides strong support for the claim that rapamycin is an effective life extension drug based on how it affects the genes associated with maximum lifespan.

Interventions that regulate genes correlated with MLS

MLS=Maximum Life Span

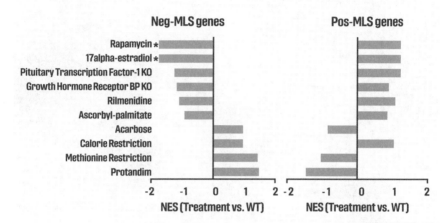

This chart shows the results from Professor Gorbunova's study on how rapamycin and nine other life extension therapies influence the genes that regulate maximum lifespan (MLS) in mammals.

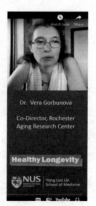

This slide was part of a webinar presentation Professor Gorbunova gave titled *From Long-Lived Animal Species to Human Interventions*. The hour-long webinar was hosted by Brian Kennedy and the National University of Singapore/ Yong Loo Lin School of Medicine's *Healthy Longevity* webinar series. To watch this entire webinar presentation by Professor Gorbunova, simply do a web search for: **"Vera Gorbunova YouTube"**

CHAPTER THREE

Rapamycin's Mechanism of Action

Rapamune (generic name sirolimus) is the brand name for rapamycin. Rapamycin is owned by Pfizer and distributed by Wyeth Pharmaceuticals LLC, which is a subsidiary of Pfizer, Inc.

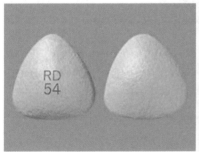 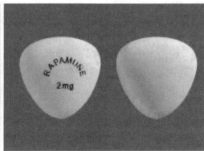

Sirolimus 2 mg tablets   Rapamune 2 mg tablets

Research efforts to understand rapamycin's mechanism of action has resulted in a critically important discovery: the links between rapamycin, mTOR and autophagy. If fact, the inextricable link between rapamycin, mTOR and autophagy explains a fundamental concept, which is what happens biochemically when not eating. What happens at the cellular level during eating (when nutrients are available) vs periods of not eating (fasting) are critically important processes that regulate health and the aging process. I'll start by discussing rapamycin, mTOR and autophagy individually.

RAPAMYCIN

Rapamycin mimics calorie restriction.[18] Animal studies in species ranging from yeasts, worms, fruit flies, spiders, fish, rodents, dogs and rhesus monkeys have reported that significantly restricting calorie intake **while maintaining adequate nutrition,** results in significant health benefits and extends both mean and maximum lifespan[19] For example, long-term calorie-restriction studies, which administer a diet that has a reduced calorie content while avoiding malnutrition, have been shown to extend the life of laboratory rats by approximately 25%.[20]

The mechanism of *how* rapamycin mimics calorie restriction has been an emerging scientific story over the past several decades. Rapamycin functions by binding to, and thereby inhibiting, the function of an intracellular enzyme named mTOR, which stands for the *mechanistic Target of Rapamycin*. This is a relatively new area of science as the mTOR signaling pathway was first discovered by multiple investigators in 1994.[21-23] However, over the past decade, more than 5,000 scientific papers have been published on mTOR.

mTOR is a fundamental regulator of cellular metabolism. Fully explaining mTOR would require a lengthy exploration into complex biochemistry, which is beyond the scope of this book. Hence, I will endeavor to explain the basic concepts without going into a biochemical quagmire. In general, rapamycin's primary benefit is that it binds to mTOR, thus partially inhibiting the activity of mTOR.

mTOR: a Key Modulator of Lifespan, Aging & the Onset of Age-Related Disease

As an enzyme, mTOR initiates the detoxification process in all cells. What's more, mTOR and the mTOR signaling pathway regulate many important cellular processes involved with protein synthesis, cellular growth, and metabolism. mTOR monitors the availability of nutrients within cells. When nutrients are available, mTOR turns on cellular metabolism, which activates anabolic (building) processes of cellular growth and proliferation. Conversely, when nutrients are scarce, mTOR is inhibited. This stops the cellular metabolic building process, which enables the body's cellular repair and regeneration processes to proceed.

Here is a somewhat simplified explanation of cellular metabolism. There are two basic metabolic modes of activity in cells throughout the body: ON and OFF. Cellular metabolism and growth are regulated by the mTOR signaling pathway. When nutrients and energy are available, mTOR turns cellular metabolism ON, which enables cells to use available nutrients and energy to build new proteins, make new cellular components, and enable cellular reproduction, also known as proliferation.

Conversely, when nutrients are not available (or are in short supply), mTOR is inhibited. This switches the body's cellular metabolism to OFF, facilitating the acti-

THE DEADLY EFFECT OF mTOR SYNDROME

The overexpression of mTOR increases the risk for cancer, diabetes, atherosclerosis, and dementia. In fact, studies in animal models suggest that the constant overexpression of mTOR is associated with accelerated onset of virtually all age-related diseases. *mTOR Syndrome* is likely a key factor related to the epidemic of chronic diseases that seem to be increasing in most countries throughout the world. This explains the importance of intermittent fasting, time restricted eating and taking rapamycin, all of which partially inhibit mTOR and promote autophagy.

vation of autophagy, which initiates the body's cellular processes of repair[24] and regeneration.[25] Autophagy has been referred to as "cellular housekeeping."[26]

During autophagy, cells remove damaged proteins, other damaged cellular components, and metabolic waste products. For example, old and damaged proteins are broken down into individual amino acids, which can be recycled and reused to rebuild and regenerate newer, healthier cellular components to replace the older damaged structures. Another way to express mTOR signaling is GROW and REST. When nutrients are available to cells, mTOR sends the GROW signal. When nutrients are in short supply, such as during a period of not eating or fasting (explained in Chapter 5), cellular metabolism switches to REST, which enables the process of autophagy to begin.

Autophagy: Cellular Detoxification & Trash Removal

In 2016, Japanese scientist Yoshinori Ohsumi was awarded the Nobel Prize in physiology and medicine for discovering the mechanism of autophagy.[24] Autophagy is one of the primary ways that cells clean up and remove their trash. Over time, various cellular components become damaged, break down, and become dysfunctional. If these waste products were allowed to build up, the cell(s) would die.[25] Thus, autophagy functions as the cellular trash collector. It initiates the process of breaking down damaged and dysfunctional cellular components for removal or recycling.

Autophagy Regulates Cellular Detoxification

Trash removal is important. Imagine mounds of trash accumulating in your kitchen, attracting pests, and allowing bacteria and mold to grow. Your living environment would soon become toxic and unlivable. A similar situation exists within cells. Autophagy MUST be activated regularly in order to keep cells clean and functioning well.

Proteins

Much of the activity of autophagy has to do with the recycling of proteins. Proteins are large complex molecules that do most of the work in cells; they play essential roles in the structure and function of all cells, tissues, and organs. Proteins are made up of many amino acids linked together. There are 20 different amino acids, which can be connected in different lengths, combinations, and shapes. Estimates suggest that the human body contains between 40,000 to 100,000 different proteins.

The shape of a protein is critical to its function. Here is a visualization experiment to help gain a better understanding of proteins. Cut three different lengths of string: 1 foot, 3 feet and 12 feet long. Now crumple each length in your hands into a ball and toss it onto a flat surface and imagine when it lands, it maintains its three-dimensional shape. Chemical bonds at different positions are what hold proteins in their three-dimensional shape.

Shape is the 'language' of proteins, like a key in a lock or a hand in a glove. But, over time, some of the structural bonds in proteins break, which cause proteins to lose their shape. Stresses like heat, acidity, and free radicals cause proteins to become misfolded and therefore non-functional.

> Shape is the 'language' of proteins, like a key in a lock or a hand in a glove.

The body is able to recognize and select damaged proteins and other injured cellular components for breakdown and recycling or removal. This process is critically important for your health. Nutrient deprivation is one of the primary mechanisms that activate cellular autophagy.[26] While autophagy can also be activated by hypoxia (lack of oxygen) or by oxidative stress, the availability and timing of nutrient delivery is the primary mechanism of autophagy that humans can control.[27,28]

And again, I want to emphasize that one way to turn on autophagy is to refrain from ingesting nutrients (food) for a period of time. When nutrients become unavailable at the cellular level, mTOR is inhibited, which enables autophagy to begin the process of cellular detoxification, waste removal and recycling.[29] Hopefully, the previous explanations enable you to understand how important regular periods of autophagy are to keep cellular biochemistry functioning properly.

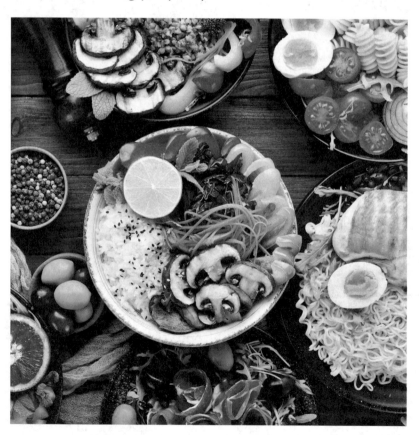

mTOR vs Autophagy: A Landmark Breakthrough in Understanding Health & Aging

After the discovery of rapamycin, subsequent research revealed that rapamycin's benefits are due to its ability to bind with mTOR. When mTOR is inhibited, this enables autophagy to proceed.[30]

Yoshinori Ohsumi made the following comment during his lecture on December 7, 2016, in Stockholm when he accepted his Nobel Prize. In his presentation, he emphasized that all living things go through what he called *"a state of relentless and ephemeral flux"* and that *"life is an equilibrium state between synthesis and degradation of old, damaged proteins."*

mTOR initiates and regulates synthesis of proteins whereas autophagy initiates and regulates the process of degradation of proteins.

Dr. Ohsumi also stated that *"recycling is essential for life."*

> mTOR initiates and regulates synthesis of proteins whereas autophagy initiates and regulates the process of degradation of old, damaged proteins.

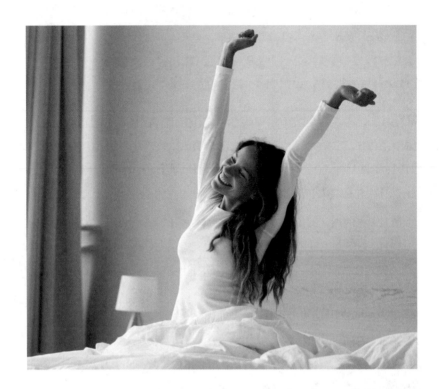

GROWTH and REST: Both these states are critical for health and life; they must be in balance. However, during the past several centuries, the processes of cellular growth vs periods of cellular rest (mTOR and autophagy) have become severely out of balance. Artificial refrigeration, which was developed in the mid-1750s, played a big role in this change because it made food easily available all the time. Consequently, humans began to eat far more frequently.

When nutrients became more readily available, cellular GROW signals started to be expressed much of the time, and time in the REST state dramatically declined. This imbalance between GROW and REST coincides with the dramatic rise in the incidence of chronic degenerative diseases that has occurred within the past several centuries. Most people eat so often that they do not spend sufficient time is the cellular REST state.

Calorie restriction and intermittent fasting were part of normal life for most people throughout thousands of years of evolution. Periods of fasting, which enable the REST state to function, are required for health. Engaging in periods of fasting are critical for healthy life extension. This is the topic of chapter 6. However, before I continue our discussion, I want to express the key topics of this book, namely rapamycin, mTOR and autophagy, in visual terms.

The mTOR/Autophagy Theory of Aging

I am proposing an *mTOR/Autophagy Theory of Aging*. It is now well established that mTOR and autophagy are fundamental mechanisms that regulate cellular metabolism, health, and the aging process itself.

Although there are many factors that influence biological aging, the mTOR/Autophagy Theory of Aging explains why these cellular mechanisms are critical factors that influence health and the aging process. The mTOR/Autophagy Theory of Aging integrates each of these processes and explains a fundamental mechanism of how the body detoxifies, recycles, and rebuilds itself throughout life.

A major cause of aging is the progressive accumulation of damaged macromolecules and components within cells. Types of damage appear as oxidized, misfolded, cross-linked, and/or aggregated proteins in cellular components, which have an abnormal structure that reduces or limits their ability to function properly. The health of an individual or organism depends on the ability to eliminate these old, dysfunctional cellular components and replace them with new, healthy cellular components. This process of degradation, recycling, protein synthesis, and renewal is regulated by autophagy and mTOR.

Humans have been evolving on Earth for several million years. Throughout most of human evolution, mTOR and autophagy were in balance. However, the mTOR/autophagy ratio is severely out of balance in the majority of people alive today, and this imbalance is one of the main reasons mankind is experiencing an epidemic of chronic degenerative diseases.

There are numerous types of dysfunction associated with aging, such as mitochondrial dysfunction, stem cell loss, cell senescence, telomere shortening, and intercellular communication decline. Within the past decade, studies have been published which have shown that autophagy is intimately involved in these mechanistic processes of aging. Thus, autophagy is increasingly being recognized as a fundamental process that can counter the effects of some of the main hallmarks of aging.[31]

Cellular components, especially proteins and enzymes, have a finite lifespan. Over time, they are exposed to external sources of stress (e.g., radiation or environmental toxins), and internal sources of stress (e.g., free radicals or oxidative stress). Autophagy is the process of breaking down, recycling and/or eliminating old, damaged cellular components. When autophagy is inhibited, the result is accelerated aging.

The Gradual Disappearance of Autophagy

Throughout most of mankind's 300,000 years of evolution, people lived as hunter-gatherers. About 12,000 years ago, the agricultural revolution resulted in a shift to farming. Growing food and livestock caused major changes in both lifestyle and food consumption.

Starting in the 1950s, Americans fell in love with household refrigerators and freezers, and the rapid acceptance of these appliances made food storable and accessible in everyone's home. More recently, technological advances in food processing, preservation, and packaging have contributed to a revolution in eating patterns in the United States and increasingly throughout the rest of the world.

Now, food is easily available all of the time. Consequently, people alive today spend much more time eating and consuming much more food compared to our ancient ancestors. Thus, mTOR is constantly being engaged and autophagy is severely under-activated.

The main goals of this book and the *mTOR/Autophagy Theory of Aging* are:

1) To educate people about rapamycin and explain its mechanism of action that enables it to increase health-span and lifespan.

2) To discuss the fundamental importance of mTOR and autophagy and explain how these mechanisms regulate cellular metabolism, health, and the aging process of all living organisms, especially humans.

3) To explain how and why the mTOR/autophagy ratio have gotten so out of balance, and how this problem is related to virtually all health problems.

4) To emphasize how rapamycin, intermittent fasting, and exercise are ways that people can correct the dysfunctional mTOR/autophagy ratio. This will increase healthspan and lifespan.

Everyone deserves to enjoy good health and achieve healthy longevity.

CHAPTER FOUR

The Rapamycin/mTOR/ Autophagy Story

Throughout my career, I've periodically created what I call "visualization experiments," which help me explain complex scientific information so that non-scientific people can easily grasp the concept. The following images will help explain the complex cellular biochemistry related to rapamycin, mTOR, and autophagy, which are key regulators of health and aging.

Ancient humans have been evolving on earth for approximately 2,000,000 years. For over 99% of this time, humans lived as hunter-gathers. Hence, I think it is safe to assume that early humans did not eat 3 meals per day. Two major factors that quickly changed human eating patterns were the development of refrigeration in the 1750s and the emergence of food processing between 1910 and 1950. When food became storable and more readily available, people began to eat more frequently and gradually began consuming larger quantities of food.

mTOR is activated when nutrients are available; autophagy is activated during the fasting state. For 99.9% of human evolution, periods of eating (mTOR activation) vs fasting (activation of autophagy) have been in a state of equilibrium that promotes health. Equilibrium doesn't mean equal parts or equal time, as in 50/50. Equilibrium refers to the amount of time that counter-balancing activities are engaged for optimal functioning of the system.

Let me use the human gut microbiome as an analogy. Approximately 100 trillion bacteria reside in the human intestinal tract. When people are healthy, approximately 85–90% microbiome consists of beneficial bacteria, called probiotics, which promote health. The other 10–15% are commensals (bacteria that are present but do no harm). We all harbor bacteria that are potential pathogens, but they generally don't cause problems unless the microbiome becomes unbalanced—too many "bad guys"

> mTOR is activated when nutrients are available; autophagy is activated during the fasting state.

and/or not enough "friendly" bacteria. However, when people take antibiotics, acid-suppressing drugs, or consume sugar or diets lacking in fiber, the microbiome gets upset, unbalanced, and health problems result.

A similar situation exists with the mTOR/Autophagy system. While the following percentages cannot be scientifically verified, I'm suggesting that the balance or equilibrium state that promotes health is about 15% mTOR activation vs 85% of time in autophagy. The following images show how the mTOR/Autophagy system in most humans has become seriously unbalanced or out of equilibrium, with disastrous health consequences. The goal of this book is to educate people about mTOR and autophagy and teach people how rapamycin can help reestablish equilibrium in the mTOR/Autophagy system and improve health.

> The goal of this book is to educate people about mTOR and autophagy and teach people how rapamycin can help reestablish mTOR/autophagy equilibrium.

The availability of nutrients and energy is what regulates the "switch" between mTOR and autophagy.[32] For hundreds of thousands of years, mTOR and autophagy were roughly in balance when people ingested and digested food during approximately 4 hours/day and remained without food for approximately 20 hours/day.

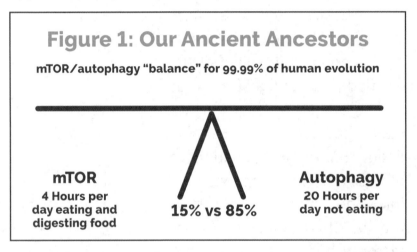

Figure 1: Our Ancient Ancestors

mTOR/autophagy "balance" for 99.99% of human evolution

mTOR
4 Hours per day eating and digesting food

15% vs 85%

Autophagy
20 Hours per day not eating

The next image (Figure 2) shows what happened to the mTOR/autophagy "balance" when food became readily available. On average, people began eating breakfast around 7 AM, followed by lunch, dinner, between-meal snacks, after-dinner desserts, and maybe an evening cocktail or a bedtime snack. On average, this meant that nutrients were available to cells in the body from 7 AM until 9 PM, or 14 hours/day, leaving only about 10 hours/day when nutrients are not available.

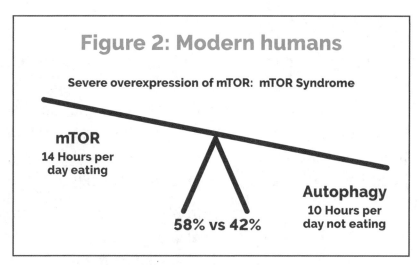

It is estimated that there are thousands of mTOR receptor in all cells. Rapamycin binds to some of the mTOR sites within cells. This partially inhibits mTOR, which reduces the amount of mTOR activity, thus increasing the time autophagy is able to function. By inhibiting mTOR, rapamycin helps bring the mTOR/Autophagy system back into balance.

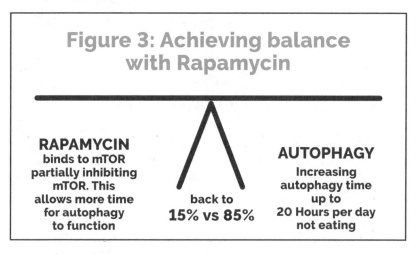

Conserved Traits

In biology, a conserved trait refers to a gene, or genes, that code for a cellular function that has existed unchanged over long periods of time. Essentially, conserved traits are genetic instructions for functions that are fundamentally important for the health and survival of an organism or species.

> The genes that regulate mTOR & autophagy were present in single cell organisms when life began to emerge on Earth approximately 3.5 billion years ago.

Autophagy[33] and mTOR[34] are conserved traits. The genes that regulate these functions are known to have been present in the first single cell organisms approximately 3.5 billion years ago. These functions have been regulating the health and longevity of cells and organisms since the beginning of life on earth.[35]

So, the mTOR/autophagy "system" has been a fundamental process that regulates the health and life of every cell since life started to evolve on earth. Yet, we humans are just learning about this critical mechanism, which is a fundamental *Rule of Health* that regulates health and our aging process.

The good news is that this is actionable, it is something we can regulate and control to improve our health and longevity. Most people suffer from some degree of mTOR Syndrome. Rapamycin can help rebalance your mTOR/autophagy system.

I hope these above images help you understand the Rapamycin/mTOR/Autophagy story.

CHAPTER FIVE

Calorie Restriction and Intermittent Fasting

Calorie restriction involves reducing the average daily intake of calories, while fasting protocols primarily focus on the frequency of eating. Fasting diets may or may not involve a reduction of caloric intake during non-fasting periods. This chapter covers calorie restriction and intermittent fasting. These topics directly relate to rapamycin and life extension because rapamycin mimics calorie restriction.

Calorie Restriction

The first animal studies reporting that calorie-restricted diets resulted in life extension were published in the 1930s. Since that time, many studies have been conducted, showing that, on average, significant calorie restriction **while maintaining adequate nutrition**, can produce increases in lifespan of 14–45% in rats and from 4–27% in mice.[36] Now, over 75 years of research has shown that calorie restriction, without malnutrition, results in significant health benefits and life extension. These effects have been

RAPAMYCIN & WEIGHT LOSS

The over expression of mTOR, which I've named mTOR Syndrome, causes insulin resistance, metabolic syndrome and increased incidence of type 2 diabetes, as well as increased inflammation and obesity.

Several studies in mice have reported that rapamycin has an anti-obesity effect. In one study, 2-month-old mice were divided into 2 groups: rapamycin & placebo controls. The db/db strain of mice, which are bred to spontaneously develop type 2 diabetes and obesity at a young age, were used in this study. After 6 months of treatment, the rapamycin-fed mice had gained 58% less body weight and 33% less fat mass compared to the mice not treated with rapamycin.

Deepa SS, et al. Rapamycin Modulates Markers of Mitochondrial Biogenesis and Fatty Acid Oxidation in the Adipose Tissue of db/db Mice. *J Biochem Pharmacol Res.* 2013 Jun;1(2):114-123.

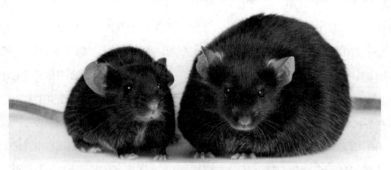

normal mouse   **db/db strain of mice develop obesity and diabetes at a young age**

shown in the following species: yeasts, worms, fruit flies, spiders, fish, rodents (hamsters, mice, and rats), dogs and monkeys.[37,38] However, it is important to realize that most humans are not willing to commit to long-term caloric restriction diets. Most people end up regaining most of the weight they initially lost.[39]

Eating: Timing (When You Eat) vs What or How Much You Eat

Over the past several decades, a great deal of research has been published regarding the timing of when we eat. During hundreds of thousands of years of human evolution, people probably did not eat 3 meals per day.

During 99.9% of human evolution, when people awoke, they did not walk into the kitchen, open the refrigerator, and pull out the milk to fix themselves a bowl of cereal. For thousands of years, most humans spent significant periods of time without eating between their cycles of eating. Hence, most people engaged in intermittent fasting throughout their lives.

Intermittent Fasting (IF)

Intermittent fasting, which is also referred to as *time-restricted eating*, is a very popular health and fitness trend that involves alternating cycles of fasting and eating. Intermittent fasting doesn't dictate calorie restriction or what type of foods you should eat, it just suggests going for longer periods of time without eating. Intermittent fasting is really an umbrella term that encompasses many variations on the timing of when to eat vs fasting time periods. There are many different protocols for intermittent fasting and there is no best fasting protocol. It is more about personal preference and finding a protocol that works for you. The most common fasting protocols are the following:

- **Time-restricted eating:** meals are consumed within a limited number of hours (6 or 8 hours), with no food consumed during the other hours of the day. Example: 16/8 Protocol—daily calories consumed within 8 consecutive hours followed by 16 hours of fasting.

- **Alternate-day fasting:** eating normally every other day, alternating with no calories or minimal calorie intake on the alternate days.

- **5:2 protocol:** eating normally for 5 days per week with 2 days per week of reduced caloric intake.

Intermittent Fasting & Weight Loss

One of the potential benefits of calorie restriction and intermittent fasting protocols is weight loss. Virtually any intermittent fasting regimen can result in some weight loss. In a review of intermittent fasting intervention trials, participants in 11 of 13 clinical trials reported varying degrees of weight loss.[40]

Rapamycin inhibits mTOR, which mimics calorie restriction, or the fasting state. This enables autophagy, or the REST state, to begin to function at the cellular level. Autophagy is dangerously absent in the lifestyle of most humans today compared with our ancestors. Healthy longevity and life extension require periods of calorie restriction and fasting. This is what rapamycin can do for you.

These days many people eat three meals per day, have occasional between-meal snacks, and following dinner, they might have dessert and an after-dinner cocktail or evening glass of beer or wine. Many people

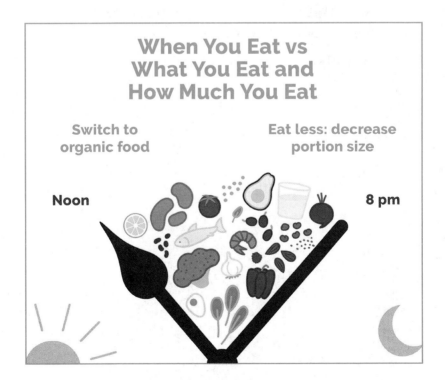

When You Eat vs What You Eat and How Much You Eat

Switch to organic food

Eat less: decrease portion size

Noon

8 pm

are consuming food periodically from 7 AM until 9 PM. That equates to 14 hours of food intake and only **10 hours of fasting** (from 9 PM until 7 AM the following morning).

I'm suggesting that for thousands of years of evolution, most people ate only once or twice per day, which is about 4 hours of eating and **20 hours of fasting**. Thus, our ancestors spent approximately twice as much time in autophagy than modern humans.

I think dysregulation of autophagy has been a significant contributor to the astronomical increase in chronic degenerative diseases over the past several centuries.[41] This is where rapamycin can help because it mimics calorie restriction or fasting, which allows autophagy to function.

CHAPTER SIX

Sarcopenia: The Importance of Weight Training, Dietary Protein, and Rapamycin

In 2017, the CDC officially recognized sarcopenia as a reportable medical condition in the new ICD-10 with the code M62.84.[42] Sarcopenia has been called a geriatric pandemic, and some experts predict that the incidence of sarcopenia could reach 40–50% among nursing home residents.[43]

Sarcopenia refers to the gradual loss of muscle mass and function with aging. The term was coined by Irwin Rosenberg in 1989.[44] Sarcopenia is now recognized as a major health problem in the elderly.

But let's back up so I can explain how my interest in this chapter's topics began. In 1992, I read a book written by William Evans, MD, and Irwin Rosenberg, MD, titled *Biomarkers*.[45] This book changed my life because it taught me the value of regularly engaging in some form of strength training. In fact, the authors showed that 10 of the most reliable biological markers of aging are all directly regulated by muscle mass. Strength training is the key.

I have followed the work of William Evans for decades. Evans discovered that when people of any age, and especially the elderly, engage in a strength training program, they can reverse some of the key biomarkers of aging.

In one study, Evans enrolled 10 frail, institutionalized 90-year-old volunteers and put them on a supervised eight-week high-intensity resistance training program. The gains they made were astounding. These included average strength gains of 174%, a 9% increase in average mid-thigh muscle area, and mean tandem gait speed improvement of 48%.[46] Maintaining muscle strength is one of the most important factors for healthy aging. However, results of a study conducted between 2011 and 2015 revealed that only 8.9% of Americans engage in weight lifting.[47]

The Importance of Protein

Proteins are complex molecules metaphorically known as the workhorses of the body. The job of proteins is to build or repair critical structures and functions in the body. In fact, over 90% of cellular functions throughout the body are regulated by proteins.[48]

There are approximately 20,000 different proteins in the human body. They range in length from 50 to 2,000 amino acids long, and they twist and turn into a wide variety of three-dimensional shapes.[49] Various sources of stress cause all proteins to incur damage and loss of function over time. Consequently, all proteins in the human body have a finite lifespan.

During autophagy, old and damaged proteins are targeted for degradation and renewal. When they are broken down, the individual amino acids are recycled and used to create healthy new proteins, enzymes, and cellular components. This cellular process is known as protein turnover (PTO). There is a constant process of PTO taking place in tissues throughout the body. The body's total muscle (protein) mass is regulated by the balance between muscle protein synthesis (MPS) and muscle protein breakdown (MPB).

Sarcopenia: A Geriatric Nightmare

The scientific term for age-related muscle loss is sarcopenia. It is common in the elderly, and it is a major predictor of falls, frailty, hospitalizations, and death. Muscle proteins in the body are constantly involved in a dynamic equilibrium between their respective rates of MPS and MPB. Sarcopenia develops when the rate of muscle breakdown exceeds the rate of protein synthesis, something that becomes more common as people age.[50]

In general, a progressive loss of muscle mass begins at about age 40, and the incidence increases dramatically as people age. Muscle mass represents about 40–50% of the body. However, most people lose approximately 8% of their muscle mass per decade until age 70.[51] After 70, the rate of muscle loss increases to about 15% per decade. Similarly, the loss of leg strength is about 10–15% per decade until 70 years of age. After that, the loss of leg strength reaches 25%–40%.[52]

Anabolic Resistance

Studies have determined that the primary problem with sarcopenia is not an increase in the rate of muscle protein breakdown, but rather, a decline in the body's ability to engage in muscle protein synthesis. This condition is known as anabolic resistance.[53]

Muscles in the elderly become less responsive to normal anabolic stimuli. However, studies have shown that this decline in age-related muscle protein synthesis can be compensated for by instituting appropriate dietary-protein/amino-acid nutritional supplementation and resistance exercise programs.

Elderly People Eat Less

Numerous studies have reported that elderly people consume less food, which amounts to about a 30% decline in energy intake between the ages of 20 and 80.[54] The term that describes this condition is the anorexia of aging.[55] There is a wide range of physical and psychological factors that can contribute to the anorexia of aging. Regardless of the causes, the bottom line is that most people eat less as they age, which often results in their becoming undernourished, especially in terms of protein.[56]

Increased Fidelity of Protein Synthesis Extends Lifespan

↻ **Cell Metabolism**   **November 2, 2021**

The paper's authors emphasize that the baseline rate of error in protein synthesis can be **hundreds of thousands of times** more then the DNA mutation rate. Making it a major neglected aspect of aging.

"We show that anti-aging drugs such as rapamycin, Torin1, and trametinib reduce translation errors, and that rapamycin **extends further organismal longevity** in RPS23 hyper-accuracy mutants. This implies a unified mode of action for diverse pharmacological anti-aging therapies."

https://www.cell.com/cell-metabolism/fulltext/S1550-4131(21)00417-4

Protein Malnutrition

Protein malnutrition is one of the more serious consequences of people's eating less as they age. At a time when older people need higher amounts of dietary protein to compensate for a decline in MPS, they consume less. However, numerous studies show that increasing dietary protein, or taking a protein or amino acid supplement, can increase MPS, and to some degree compensate for the age-related decline in MPS.[57,58]

The RDA for Protein Is Too Low

Recently, results from several epidemiological and clinical studies have indicated that higher protein intake for adults could result in better health outcomes. Consequently, health experts in the U.S. and Europe believe that current dietary protein recommendation of 0.8 gm/kg is too low. The consensus is that the dietary protein recommendation should be increased to between 1.0 gm and 2.0 gm/kg per day, which represents a substantial increase.[59-62]

Bottom line? Current government recommendations for the ingestion of dietary protein is set too low. This is especially problematic for the elderly who require greater amounts of daily protein to compensate for the age-associated decline in muscle protein synthesis.

Quality of Protein for Muscle Growth

Animal-based proteins are considered "complete" because they contain all the essential amino acids that humans require. Plant-based proteins (except soy), on the other hand, are "incomplete" because they lack one or more of the essential amino acids. This is one reason plant-based protein is less effective than animal protein for muscle growth. Also, plant-based proteins are less efficient at building muscle protein because they are more difficult to digest and have lower amino acid content than animal protein.[63]

Leucine is the primary amino acid that triggers mTOR in a dose-responsive manner to initiate muscle protein synthesis and muscle recovery after a workout.[64,65] The International Society of Sports Nutrition states that "acute protein doses should strive to contain 700–3000 mg of leucine and/or a higher relative leucine content, in addition to a balanced array of the essential amino acids."[66] A meta-analysis of studies in which leucine-rich protein supplements were provided to older adults with sarcopenia reported that leucine supplementation does indeed result in improved muscle strength in elderly individuals with sarcopenia.[67]

Resistance Training & Sarcopenia

Numerous studies have identified resistance training as a highly effective intervention to prevent and treat sarcopenia. Indeed, resistance training has been shown to be the *most effective* modality to increase muscle mass and strength in elderly individuals.[68] A meta-analysis of 14 studies revealed the following conclusions: older people who engage in resistance training experience a decline in body fat mass, and increases in handgrip strength, knee extension strength, gait speed, and the Timed Up and Go walking test.[69]

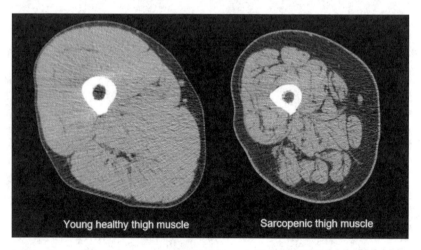

Young healthy thigh muscle   Sarcopenic thigh muscle

Timing of Protein/Leucine Intake for Maximum Benefit

Strength or resistance training stimulates muscle protein synthesis by sensitizing muscles to the anabolic effects of insulin and amino acid nutrients, especially leucine. Resistance training stimulates both MPS and MPB. However, the stimulation of MPS is greater than the stimulation of MPB. Therefore, resistance exercise does not cause a loss of muscle.[70]

Studies have shown that protein supplementation, before and/or after workouts, promotes an increase in physical performance, training session recovery, lean body mass, muscle mass, and strength. However, the gains differ based on the type and amount of protein utilized.

Following the consumption of protein, MPS is increased for about three hours, with a peak occurring at about 45–90 minutes. After three hours, MPS reverts to baseline, even though serum amino acid levels remain elevated.[71]

Protein quality is especially important for the elderly in their efforts to maintain muscle mass or minimize the loss of muscle mass as they age. Factors that influence protein quality include digestibility and amino acid content. Whey protein is a very high-quality protein because it contains a high amount of leucine. It is also easily digested and absorbed. Whey protein has been shown to stimulate muscle protein synthesis more effectively than casein or soy protein.

Studies consistently show that protein ingestion following an episode of strength training stimulates muscle protein synthesis for up to three hours. Consequently, ingesting protein or amino acids supplements directly after episodes of resistance exercise will optimize muscle protein synthesis.[72] Also, some carbohydrate should be consumed along with the protein because leucine stimulates muscle protein synthesis more effectively in the presence of insulin.[73]

Autophagy: Rapamycin & Protein Recycling

As discussed earlier, autophagy is the process that regulates protein turnover and recycling. Nutrient activation of mTOR results in protein synthesis and muscle growth. However, constant overexpression of mTOR, which I refer to as *mTOR Syndrome*, is somewhat like driving your car with the accelerator pushed to the floor constantly. This leads to many health problems, such as cancer, cardiovascular disease, and diabetes, to name a few.

When people engage in activities that activate autophagy, such as taking rapamycin, exercising, or intermittent fasting, it is important to address the quality, the timing, and the amount of protein being ingested. Breaking a period of fasting with the ingestion of high-quality protein will optimize muscle protein synthesis when mTOR is reactivated.

Rapamycin Reduces Errors in Protein Translation

DNA is stationary within the nucleus of cells, but proteins move. As I mentioned previously, proteins are the workhorses in cells, doing the work of building or repairing and rebuilding the body. However, errors frequently occur during protein synthesis, which can result in misfolded and dysfunctional proteins.

> In a recently published paper, it was reported that rapamycin reduces protein translation errors.

DNA mutations contribute to a wide range of diseases and have long been associated with accelerated biological aging. However, in recent years, it has become apparent that the rate of error in protein synthesis or protein translation may be hundreds of thousands of times more frequent than the rates of DNA mutations.

A recently published paper reported that rapamycin reduces protein translation errors. This is an exciting new area of research because it presents another way that rapamycin improves health and extends lifespan. This mechanism is independent of rapamycin's effect on mTOR and autophagy.[74]

Summary

High-quality protein consumption, especially leucine, is important in order to optimize muscle protein synthesis. This is crucial for older individuals, especially those engaging in strength training, and particularly for people engaging in rapamycin therapy.

CHAPTER SEVEN
Summary of Rapamycin's Health Benefits

Scientific interest in rapamycin and mTOR-inhibiting drugs is exploding. For example, from 1975 to 2008, there were about 10 articles or studies per year published on rapamycin and aging.

From 2009 to 2016 there were an average of 180 articles or studies per year published on rapamycin and aging.

A PubMed search I conducted on February 24, 2023, revealed 6,695 publications with the word rapamycin in the title, and there were 35,541 listings with rapamycin in the title or abstract.

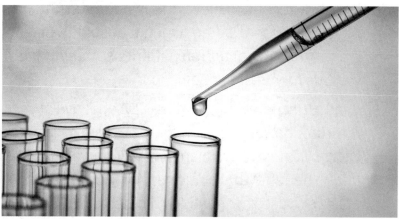

However, at the time of this writing, very few human clinical trials have been conducted to evaluate the potential health benefits from rapamycin, or other rapalogs, at doses that achieve partial inhibition of mTOR (rapalogs are synthetic drugs that are analogues of rapamycin).

The reasons for the scarcity of the type of scientific studies that are needed include:

> The majority of studies conducted to date are animal studies.

a. The majority of studies conducted to date are animal studies. Some of this information is useful. However, the digestive and immune systems of animals are quite different from those of humans.

b. Most of the human clinical trials conducted have been administering daily—not weekly—doses to prevent organ rejection for patients who had previously received an organ transplant, or as a chemotherapy drug for patients suffering from various forms of cancer.

c. Because rapamycin's original FDA approvals were for immune suppression and as a form of chemotherapy, most physicians were unaware of the health benefits that could result when prescribed at lower doses for partial inhibition of mTOR.

As you will learn throughout this book, studies show that using once-a-week dosing with 5–10 mg of rapamycin does not appear to suppress immune function compared to the daily-dosing protocols when rapamycin is used in chemotherapy or for immune suppression.[75]

One of the primary goals of this book is to educate physicians about mTOR Syndrome and the health benefits that result from partial inhibition of mTOR.

What Illnesses Can Benefit from Rapamycin?

I believe that the vast majority of health problems will respond favorably to rapamycin therapy at doses that partially inhibit mTOR. I think most cellular and biochemical processes that are out of balance can improve with rapamycin therapy. On the other hand, if someone already has a weakened artery, rapamycin probably won't prevent it from rupturing at some future date. If an individual has bone-on-bone osteoarthritis, rapamycin won't regrow cartilage. In short, rapamycin is not going to help with everyone's health problems.

However, mTOR and autophagy are a counter-regulatory system that is a fundamental regulator of cellular biochemistry. This system regulates the health and the lifespan of every cell in the body. And virtually everyone is out of balance and suffering from mTOR

Syndrome. Hence, rapamycin therapy has the potential to improve overall health in a vast majority of people alive today.

In this chapter, I am going to review some studies and provide some information that shows how rapamycin therapy can provide health benefits to people suffering from some of the most common age-related diseases.

In most cases, the medical profession treats age-related diseases separately and symptomatically. There is increasing evidence that a common underlying process is involved in age-related diseases and the aging process. There is also mounting evidence suggesting that dysregulation of mTOR and autophagy within cells is a fundamental underlying mechanism of age-related diseases. In fact, the mechanistic Target of Rapamycin, or mTOR, has been referred to as *"The Grand ConducTOR of Metabolism and Aging".*[76]

This chapter is devoted to showing how rapamycin can reduce the risks or delay the onset of age-related diseases, and be used as a treatment for them.

RAPAMYCIN & CANCER

Studies have shown that the mechanistic Target of Rapamycin (mTOR) and mTOR signaling pathways regulate many aspects of cancer metabolism and tumor growth. Rapamycin is a prime candidate to slow the progression of cancer because by inhibiting mTOR, it inhibits cellular growth and proliferation.

The overexpression of mTOR, or mTOR Syndrome, is linked to tumor growth in multiple types of cancer.[77] Consequently, mTOR inhibiting drugs such as rapamycin and various rapalogs (synthetic derivatives of rapamycin) have attracted attention as potential anti-cancer agents for a number of different types of cancer.

Everolimus and temsirolimus have been FDA-approved for the treatment of renal cell carcinoma. Temsirolimus is also approved for the treatment of mantle cell lymphoma, which is a type of non-Hodgkin

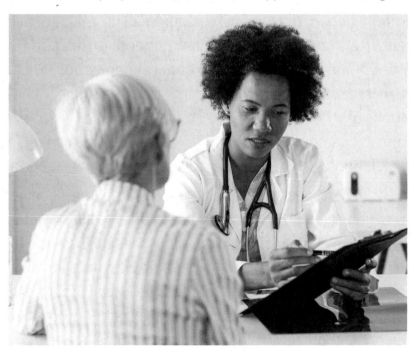

lymphoma that develops in middle-aged and older adults. In addition to these drugs, rapamycin (sirolimus) and ridaforolimus (formerly named deforolimus) are currently being evaluated in clinical trials on various types of cancer.[78]

Studies suggest that mTOR inhibitors suppress tumor growth by halting cellular proliferation in tumors, accelerating the death of tumor cells, and suppressing a tumor's ability to build new blood vessels (angiogenesis), which inhibits the tumor's growth.[79]

Studies have revealed that organ transplant recipients have a much higher likelihood of developing cancer. In fact, cancer has become the leading cause of death among organ transplant recipients. The incidence of cancer among organ transplant patients is three to five times higher than that of the general population, with a correspondingly poorer outcome in late-stage cancer.[80] Much of the information regarding rapamycin and cancer has come from data following organ transplant recipients taking rapamycin to prevent organ rejection.

In 2019 in the United States, 39,717 people received an organ transplant. Kidney transplants were the most common (23,401) followed by liver transplants (8,896), heart (3,551), and lung (2,714).[81] People who have received an organ transplant need to continually take drugs that suppress the immune system to prevent their body from rejecting their new organ. However, these drugs come with their own long list of potential side effects. One of the major side effects is the increased incidence of cancer.

Organ transplant recipients often develop multiple, very aggressive nonmelanoma skin cancers. Surgery is frequently not a good option for patients who develop these multiple nonmelanoma skin cancers.[82] Results from five clinical trials show that switching the immunosuppressive drug therapy to rapamycin/sirolimus, or another mTOR inhibitor named everolimus, results in a reduction in the development nonmelanoma skin cancers.[83]

A search on *ClinicalTrials.gov* website on February 18, 2023, using the search terms *rapamycin* and *cancer* revealed that there currently hundreds of clinical cancer trials being conducted using either rapamycin or other rapalogs. Many of the trials are using just one drug, while many other trials are using rapamycin or one of the rapalogs in combination with other chemotherapy agents.

RAPAMYCIN & CARDIOVASCULAR DISEASE

Rapamycin/Sirolimus-impregnated stents prevent stent restenosis.

In 1977, the balloon angioplasty procedure was introduced, which quickly became a revolution in interventional cardiology. Balloon angioplasty is a minimally invasive surgical procedure that widens arteries or veins that have become narrowed or obstructed by plaque deposits. In this procedure, a deflated balloon is guided into the constricted area of the vessel and then inflated. This expands the constricted area in the blood vessel, which improves blood flow. However, many patients experience restenosis (re-narrowing) within three to six months following the initial balloon angioplasty procedure.

In April 2003, a new revolution in interventional cardiology began following the FDA's approval of stents containing synthetic polymers impregnated with sirolimus. The stent gradually releases sirolimus, which inhibits smooth muscle proliferation and subsequent re-narrowing of the blood vessel.

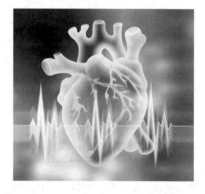

More than two million stents are implanted every year in the United States. Of these, approximately 1.2 million are coronary stents. Over the past two decades, there have been improvements in stents and their drug-releasing polymers. Owing to better outcomes, stents containing sirolimus or other "sirolimus analogues" have become cardiologists' leading choice for these lifesaving procedures.[85]

Beyond stents, the use of rapamycin as an overall treatment for cardiovascular disease is also garnering interest. Heart attacks and strokes are still the main causes of death in the United States, and cardiovascular risks generally increase as people age. Over time, arteries become more susceptible to plaque buildup, scarring, elasticity loss, and increasing stiffness. Many factors contribute to arterial damage, such as environmental toxins, elevated blood sugar, oxidative stress, and inflammation.

As I emphasize throughout this book, most people suffer from constant mTOR activation, which I call mTOR Syndrome. Aging arteries suffer from overactivation of mTOR, but studies have shown this can be reversed with rapamycin. In 2017, results of a study published in the journal *Aging Cell* reported that rapamycin therapy successfully reversed arterial aging in mice. While aging results in increased stiffness in large arteries such as the aorta, rapamycin treatment successfully reduced aortic stiffness. It was proposed that these improvements are due to decreases in oxidative stress and glycation, and the activation of AMPK. Rapamycin's ability to reduce oxidative stress within the artery wall resulted in improved arterial dilation and increased blood flow.[86]

Stresses on the heart, such as elevated blood pressure, diminished blood supply and oxygen, and oxidative stress cause the heart to work harder. Over time, this results in an enlargement of the heart (called cardiac hypertrophy), which frequently progresses to heart failure and is considered to be a risk factor for cardiovascular disease and death.[87] It has now been shown that rapamycin-induced mTOR suppression and autophagy activation inhibit the development of cardiac hypertrophy.[88]

Another study reported that rapamycin protects heart cells and improves cardiac function by activating autophagy in cardiomyocytes (heart cells). This, in turn, reduces the risk of chronic heart failure.[89]

Thus far, most of the studies on rapamycin and cardiovascular diseases have been conducted in animal models. However, ClinicalTrials.gov shows that several human clinical trials are under way.

RAPAMYCIN & PARKINSON'S DISEASE

STUDY: Neuroprotective effect of rapamycin against Parkinson's disease in mice.[90]

In their conclusions, the authors state, "Rapamycin inhibits the activation of mTOR pathway, which contributes to **protect against the loss of dopaminergic neurons and provide behavioral improvements in mice with Parkinson's disease. These results are partially related to the ability of rapamycin in inducing autophagy and reducing oxidative stress.**"

RAPAMYCIN & ALZHEIMER'S DISEASE

STUDY: Inhibition of mTOR by rapamycin abolishes cognitive deficits and reduces amyloid-beta levels in a mouse model of Alzheimer's disease.[91]

The authors state in their **conclusions**: "Our data suggest that inhibition of mTOR by rapamycin, an intervention that extends lifespan in mice, can slow or block Alzheimer's disease progression in a transgenic mouse model of the disease. **Rapamycin, already used in clinical settings, may be a potentially effective therapeutic agent for the treatment of Alzheimer's disease.**"

RAPAMYCIN & MULTIPLE SCLEROSIS

STUDY: Promising effect of rapamycin on multiple sclerosis.[92]

The aim of this trial was to evaluate rapamycin's therapeutic effects on clinical and radiological aspects, regulatory T cells proliferation and FOXP3 and GARP gene expression in patients with relapsing-remitting multiple sclerosis (RRMS).

All the patients had some degree of significant reduction in mean plaque area size and minimum and maximum plaque size. Fifty percent of patients' expanded disability status scale (EDSS) scores decreased after the treatment, yet not significantly. The expression rate of FOXP3 and GARP genes in Tregs increased after the therapy. In their conclusion, the authors stated, **"We found a promising response to rapamycin among our cases with minor side effects and it may be considered as a therapeutic option of this disease."**

RAPAMYCIN & RHEUMATOID ARTHRITIS

STUDY: Low-dose sirolimus immunoregulation therapy in patients with active rheumatoid arthritis: A 24-week follow-up of the randomized, open-label, parallel-controlled trial.[93]

By 24 weeks, the patients with sirolimus experienced significant reduction in their DAS28 score, which is an assessment of disease activity (swelling and tenderness) in 28 joints throughout the body. They had a higher level of Tregs (regulatory T cells) compared with patients on conventional therapy alone, which indicates that sirolimus can partly restore the reduction in Tregs commonly seen in RDA patients. Patients taking sirolimus also reduced their usage of immunosuppressant drugs to control disease activity compared with the conventional group.

RAPAMYCIN & SYSTEMIC LUPUS ERYTHEMATOSUS (SLE)

STUDY: Improvement of renal and non-renal SLE outcome measures on sirolimus therapy— A 21-year follow-up study of 73 patients.[94]

The safety, tolerance, and outcome measures were assessed in 73 SLE patients who were treated with siro-limus for three months or longer. All patients gained increases in C3 and C4 compliment levels (C3 and C4 are proteins that are part of the immune system, which are commonly low in patients with SLE). Of the 73 patients, the following minor sides effects were reported: mouth sores (2/73), headaches (1/73), and GI discomfort (6/73). Two patients stopped taking siro-limus, one due to headaches and one due to recurrent infections. This study indicates that sirolimus is well tolerated and provides long-term therapeutic effec-tiveness in controlling manifestations of SLE.

RAPAMYCIN & WEIGHT LOSS

Obesity is now recognized as a global pandemic, with rates doubling in over 70 countries since 1980.[95] In the United States, over 70% of Americans are overweight or obese.[96] The ongoing obesity epidemic has intensi-

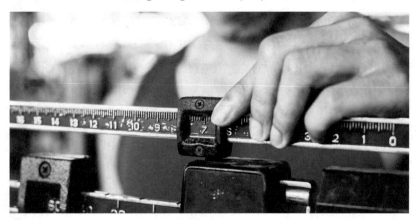

fied the search for effective methods to achieve weight loss. The obesity crisis has intensified efforts to find solutions to this problem.

Is Rapamycin a Potential Therapy for Obesity?

By inhibiting mTOR, rapamycin mimics caloric restriction. Fasting, or not eating, also inhibits mTOR. In nonhuman primates, caloric restriction and has been shown to result in loss of weight and body fat, reduced risks of cancer and cardiovascular disease, and increased lifespan.[97,98] If rapamycin's ability to inhibit mTOR and mimic calorie restriction provides similar benefits in humans, it may be a useful therapeutic tool to treat obesity.

Caloric restriction, also called dietary restriction, is one of the most common methods people use in their attempt to lose weight. Data from human clinical trials have shown that caloric restriction, without malnutrition, is one of the most successful approaches in the prevention and treatment of obesity and its complications.[99] However, studies have shown that most people find it very difficult to sustain calorie-restricted diets. Furthermore, among those who initially lose weight on these diets, most will regain it.[100]

In animal models and human clinical trials, rapamycin correlates to a decrease in food intake and an increase in weight loss.[101] Rapamycin is a drug that has been shown to promote weight loss and decrease fat mass in both animal models and humans.[102] Thus, rapamycin may provide the benefits of caloric restriction for people without requiring them to actually adhere to a calorie-restricted diet.

Rapamycin has also been shown to communicate an "excessive nutrient" signal to the hypothalamus, which triggers an anorexic response to reduce food consumption. This results in a decrease in the synthesis of leptin and a corresponding decrease in adiposity.[103] Consequently, rapamycin is increasingly being recognized as a possible treatment for obesity.

RAPAMYCIN & ANTI-INFLAMMATORY ACTIVITY

As previously mentioned, numerous studies have reported that surgical implantation of stents impregnated with rapamycin reduce inflammation, which significantly reduces re-narrowing of the affected blood vessel.[104]

A recent development in cardiology has been the rapamycin-loaded nanoparticle delivery systems that are much more effective at delivering rapamycin to inflamed blood vessels. In a mouse study, the rapamycin nanoparticles significantly reduced localized vascular inflammation within seven days. The authors of this study report that this new rapamycin nanoparticle delivery system can reverse vascular inflammation and could be a promising intervention for acute stabilization of late-stage plaques.[105]

RAPAMYCIN FOR ACTIVE UVEITIS

Uveitis is a form of eye inflammation that causes eye redness, pain, and blurred vision. If left untreated, it can result in blindness. Patients with uveitis are traditionally treated with anti-inflammatory corticosteroid drugs. When rapamycin was utilized[106] to treat patients with uveitis, corticosteroid use was either decreased or eliminated. The authors reported that rapamycin is a well tolerated and effective anti-inflammatory treatment for this condition.

RAPAMYCIN & OSTEOPOROSIS

Results of some studies suggest rapamycin may be useful for the prevention and treatment of bone problems such as osteoporosis, and the acceleration of fracture healing.[108,109] However a conflicting study published in 2021 reported that rapamycin has a negative impact on bone health. When I read the full text of this clinical trial, I realized that the mice in this study were given extremely high doses of rapamycin, relative to what is contemplated for human longevity purposes.[110] Rapamycin has already been approved to reduce bone pain in patients with bone metastases due to its ability to improve mTOR/autophagy balance, which promotes building of healthy new bone.[111] Bone loss during exposure to microgravity is a major threat to astronauts' health during space missions. This prompted NASA to fund studies on rapamycin's ability to prevent osteoporosis, not only in space, but also on Earth.[112,113]

Studies show that mTOR plays a key role in regulating bone metabolism, which sheds light on the pathogenesis of osteoporosis. In one study, rapamycin was administered to 24-month-old rats for 12 weeks.[114] The results revealed that rapamycin activated autophagy in bone cells, which reduced the severity of age-related bone changes in old male rats. It had previously been documented that the strain of rats used in this study experience age-related bone loss and decreased bone turnover comparable to that seen in elderly men, hence they were judged to be an appropriate animal for this study.[115] In their conclusions, the authors stated the following, "Therefore, rapamycin might be a feasible therapeutic approach for senile osteoporosis."[116]

In another study, the authors stated that by inhibiting mTOR and activating autophagy, treatment with rapamycin inhibited bone resorption while promoting bone formation, which helped to reduce the development of early osteoporosis in rats.[117]

RAPAMYCIN DELAYS HEARING LOSS

When rapamycin therapy is initiated in middle-aged mice (14 months old), the results revealed that rapamycin therapy decreased the onset of age-related hearing loss.[118]

Pendred syndrome is a genetic disorder that causes bilateral hearing loss in children. Children born with this disorder begin to lose their hearing at birth, or by the time they reach three years of age. This condition can also affect the thyroid gland, and it sometimes causes balance problems. The results of one study indicated that low-dose rapamycin therapy not only decreased acute symptoms but also showed the potential to prevent the progression of hearing loss in patients with Pendred syndrome.[119]

RAPAMYCIN FOR PERIODONTAL DISEASE

Periodontal disease is one of many health-related problems that increase with age. Periodontal disease is mainly caused by infections, inflammation of the gums, and oral microbiome dysbiosis. As the disease progresses, it can lead to bone and tooth loss, and it is a risk factor for systemic diseases such as cardiovascular disease, lung diseases pneumonia and COPD, and Alzheimer's disease and dementia.[120-122] Individuals with type 2 diabetes who have advanced periodontal disease have three-times greater risk of death compared to individuals with mild or no periodontal disease.[123]

Both the frequency and severity of periodontal disease increase with age, and most people over 50 are affected.[124] Because periodontal disease is easy to visualize, assess, and monitor, it is a good disease model to test the effectiveness of rapamycin to slow down the progression of aging.

In an eight-week study with elderly mice, treatment with rapamycin resulted in a rejuvenation of the aged oral cavity, including regeneration of periodontal bone, and a reduction in gingival and periodontal-bone inflammation. Rapamycin not only delayed the onset of gum disease in aged mice, but it actually reversed the progression of the disease. Rapamycin treatment also converted the oral microbiome of the elderly mice to one similar to that of young mice.[125]

Further studies are needed, but this study suggests that rapamycin holds the promise to be an effective treatment to reverse periodontal disease and improve oral health in the elderly.

RAPAMYCIN FOR MACULAR DEGENERATION

Age-related macular degeneration is the most common cause of blindness in the world. When rats were treated with rapamycin, there was a decrease in the incidence and severity of damage to the retina. Another important result was that rapamycin prevented destruction of ganglion neurons in the retina. In their closing statement, the authors stated the following: "Our data suggest the therapeutic potential of rapamycin for treatment and prevention of retinopathy."[126]

In an experimental model of age-related macular degeneration with mice,[127] treatment with rapamycin reduced inflammation and levels of oxidative stress, and protected against retinal degeneration. The benefits were found to be more significant after seven days of treatment. In their closing statement, the authors stated that this study potentially provides powerful experimental support for the use of rapamycin for the treatment of age-related macular degeneration.

RAPAMYCIN & GLAUCOMA

Glaucoma is another leading cause of blindness throughout the world. The visual impairment in glaucoma results from pressure-induced damage to retinal ganglion cells. In a study with rats afflicted with chronic ocular hypertension, treatment with rapamycin dramatically promoted the survival of the retinal ganglion cells.[128]

Glaucoma is associated with dysregulated glucose metabolism, which leads to optic nerve degenera-

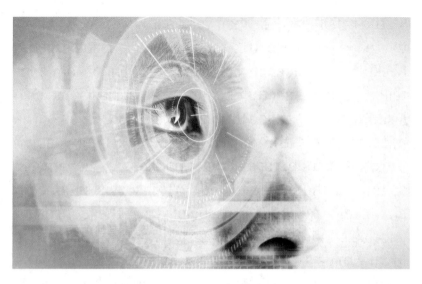

tion. In both mouse and rat models of glaucoma, administration of rapamycin actively prevented the neurodegeneration of the optic nerves caused by increased ocular pressure.[129]

TOPICAL APPLICATION OF RAPAMYCIN FOR SKIN CONDITIONS

Rapamycin has been used "off-label" to treat facial angiofibromas,[130] which are noncancerous tumors made up of blood vessels and connective tissue that usually appear as red bumps on the face, especially on the nose and cheeks. Application of a 0.4% topical rapamycin solution can provide significant improvement. One study reported that applying a compounded topical rapamycin cream resulted in dramatic improvement of facial angiofibromas.[131]

The mTOR pathway has been shown to be hyperac-
tivated in psoriasis. In a mouse study of psoriasis,the
backs of the mice were shaved and then cream containing a chemical that produces a psoriasis-like skin
irritation was applied directly to the skin.[132] Half of the
mice received the psoriasis-inducing chemical. In
the other group, researchers applied a 1% rapamycin
solution to the skin, followed by the psoriasis-inducing
chemical. The results revealed that the degree of
psoriasis inflammation was significantly less severe
in the mice treated topically with rapamycin. The
data from this study suggest that mTOR signaling is
involved in the psoriatic disease process, and that
topical application of mTOR inhibitors may become a
new approach to treating psoriasis.

In a more general sense, some experts have suggested that topical rapamycin may be useful for the
treatment of various types of skin conditions, such
as skin spots, wrinkles, and photo-aged skin. There
is also ample evidence that topical rapamycin prepa-
ration can accelerate the healing of various types of
skin wounds.[133]

RAPAMYCIN FOR MEMORY, COGNITIVE DECLINE, & BRAIN AGING

The brain is highly sensitive to mTOR. Compelling
evidence indicates that mTOR activity regulates
cognitive function. However, mTOR hyperactivity

has been shown to have harmful effects on brain function. Several studies have reported that hyperactive mTOR signaling, or what I am calling mTOR Syndrome, is associated with cognitive decline.[134,135] Some studies have also reported that overexpression of mTOR is found in the brains of patients with Alzheimer's disease.[136]

A hallmark of Alzheimer's disease is the accumulation of beta-amyloid and tau protein deposits in brain neurons. In a mouse model of Alzheimer's disease, administration of rapamycin, which reduced mTOR activity, resulted in a decline in the production of beta-amyloid and tau protein along with improvements in learning and memory function.[137]

NOT TAKING RAPAMYCIN MAY BE AS DANGEROUS AS SMOKING

The following two paragraphs are excerpted from an article by Dr. Mikhail Blagosklonny titled **"Rapamycin for Longevity"**, published in October 2019 issue of the journal *Aging*.[138]

"Strangely, the fear of tobacco smoking is less intense than the fear of rapamycin. But whereas smoking shortens both the healthspan and lifespan, rapamycin extends them. Smoking increases the incidence of cancer and other age-related diseases. Rapamycin prevents cancer in mice and humans. Heavy smoking shortens life expectancy by about

6–10 years. In other words, simply not smoking prolongs life by 6–10 years."

"In middle-aged mice, just 3 months of high-dose rapamycin treatment was sufficient to increase life expectancy up to 60%.[139] When taken late in life, rapamycin increases lifespan by 9–14%.[140] This possibly equates to more than 7 years of human life. By comparison, smokers who quit late in life (at age 65 and older), gain between 1.4 and 3.7 years.[141] Considered in those terms, one could say that in the elderly, *not* taking rapamycin may be even more 'dangerous' than smoking. Finally, rapamycin may be especially beneficial to smokers and former smokers. While the carcinogens from tobacco cause lung cancer in mice, rapamycin decreases tobacco-induced lung cancer multiplicity by 90%."

CHAPTER 8

Rapamycin Improves Reproductive Health

According to the World Health Organization, "reproductive health is a state of complete physical, mental, and social well-being and not merely the absence of disease or infirmity, in all matters relating to the reproductive system and to its functions and processes." What this means is that all people, no matter their gender or age, should be able to enjoy a satisfying sex life, and that they are able to reproduce when they desire. Yet, too often reproductive problems arise, particularly as an individual ages. However, emerging evidence suggests that rapamycin may be able effectively help both men and women maintain or regain their sexual and reproductive capacity.

Erectile Dysfunction

A significant number of men have reported experiencing an increase in the frequency of erections after they start taking rapamycin. Several animal studies have reported that rapamycin improves erectile function. As a result, an explanation of the biochemical process responsible for this occurrence is beginning to emerge.[142]

FREQUENCY OF ERECTILE DYSFUNCTION

Erectile dysfunction (ED) is a far more frequent condition than most people realize, and it often has a detrimental effect on relationships and quality of life. Data from the 2001–2002 National Health and Nutrition Examination Survey (NHANES) reported that 18.4% of men in the United States, or about 18 million, suffer from ED.[142]

There are many physical and psychological factors that can contribute to the development of ED. Numerous medical conditions can lead to ED, such as type 2 diabetes, obesity, high blood pressure, atherosclerosis, chronic kidney disease, Peyronie's disease, and injuries related to treatments for prostate cancer, including radiation therapy and prostate surgery.

The increased frequency of ED associated with these diseases is shocking. For example, in a meta-analysis of 145 studies, it was reported that 37.5% of men with Type 1 diabetes and 66.3% of men with Type 2 diabetes suffer from erectile dysfunction.[143] In another study, 79% of obese men (BMI 25 or higher) suffer from ED.[144] Approximately two-thirds of men with elevated blood pressure also have some degree of erectile dysfunction.[145]

RAPAMYCIN IMPROVES ERECTILE DYSFUNCTION

When rats with both type 1 diabetes and erectile dysfunction were treated with rapamycin, they experienced improved erectile function compared to diabetic rats that served as controls.[146] The authors stated that this is the first study to report that rapamycin, which induces autophagy, is effective at restoring erectile function in rats with diabetes. These results suggest that rapamycin may possibly be a new therapy for reversing diabetic erectile dysfunction in men as well.

MECHANISM: HOW RAPAMYCIN IMPROVES ED

In one study with rats, it was shown that rapamycin helps protect the cavernous nerve, which is the primary nerve that regulates penile erection. Following the intentional injury to the animal's cavernous nerve, erectile function returned much faster in those rats treated with rapamycin.[147]

Overactivation of mTOR, caused by far more frequent ingestion of calories compared to ancestral humans, is associated with increased production of reactive oxygen species (ROS) and damaging free radicals. In a mouse study, 90 young male mice were fed a high-fat, high-sugar Western diet for 12 weeks. For the final four weeks, half of the mice were injected with 2 mg/kg rapamycin three days per week. The other half, which was the control group, received saline injections three days per week.

At the conclusion of the study, the researchers noted that the Western diet had caused the mice to develop significant erectile dysfunction. They also concluded that the diet sparked an increase in the production of ROS (which would explain the damage to the cavernous nerve), resulting in ED. However, erectile function was restored in the mice treated with rapamycin. These mice also experienced a reduction in the activity of the enzyme NADPH oxidase, which is known to generate ROS. Thus, rapamycin therapy reduced the production of the NADPH oxidase enzyme in the penis. This, in turn, led to a reduction in damage to the cavernous nerve in the penis and improved erectile function.[148]

> Researchers noted that the Western diet had caused the mice to develop significant erectile dysfunction.

The results of this experiment in mice, in which rapamycin helped prevent damage to the cavernous nerve in the penis, may explain why some men experience improved erectile function after starting to take rapamycin.

Rapamycin Extends Female Fertility

Women's peak reproductive years typically last from their late teens into their late 20s. Around age 30, fertility (the ability to get pregnant) begins to decline. This decline accelerates once women reach their midthirties and by age 45, fertility has declined to the point that most women are not able to become pregnant. Also, becoming pregnant after age 35 is associated with increased risks of premature birth and birth defects.[149]

These days, however, many women are choosing to delay having children until their late 30s or 40s. Two common reasons for this shift are a woman's desire to establish a career or wait until she is financially secure. Also, many women say they delay starting a family because they have not found the right partner yet.

RAPAMYCIN KEEPS THE REPRODUCTIVE CLOCK TICKING

mTOR regulates cellular metabolism, which in turn, controls all biological activities. Recently, studies have shown that mTOR plays a role in regulating many aspects of the female reproductive cycle, including the development of ovarian follicles, the maturation of oocytes, the onset of puberty, and ovarian aging.[150-153]

Age-related ovarian failure in women cannot be reversed. However, results from several animal studies suggest that rapamycin may extend a woman's reproductive years. In one animal experiment, rapamycin was given for two weeks (considered short-term treatment) to 8-week-old mice (equivalent to 20- to 30-year-old humans) and to 8-month-old mice (equivalent to 38- to 47-year-old humans). The short-term treatment caused some mild disturbances in ovarian function for up to two months following the two weeks of treatment. However, in the long-term, two weeks of rapamycin treatment preserved immature ovarian follicles, improved the overall micro-environment in the ovaries, and increased the quality and yield of oocytes. This resulted in an increase in the number of pups per litter in both the young and old treatment groups for up to 16 months.[154]

RAPAMYCIN MAY DELAY MENOPAUSE

Because rapamycin has the potential to extend fertility, there is some speculation that it may also help delay the onset of menopause. This is likely due to the drug's ability to inhibit mTOR signaling, which, in turn, prolongs ovarian function and the length of the female reproductive lifespan.

During one placebo-controlled animal study, adult female rats were injected with rapamycin (5 mg/kg) every other day for 10 weeks. This effectively inhibited mTOR signaling and resulted in a two-fold increase in the number of primordial ovarian follicles.[199] This suggests that, as a natural consequence of extending fertility, rapamycin may also delay menopause. Although more research is needed, this delay could have a positive impact on women over the age of 50 by reducing the risk of menopause-related diseases like cardiovascular disease and osteoporosis. In their concluding statement, the authors of this study state, "We optimistically consider that rapamycin or its derivatives could be used as an effective drug for preventing premature ovarian failure and delaying the onset of menopause in obese or even healthy women in the future."

CHAPTER NINE

Rapamycin's Safety Profile

At the doses used for life extension, rapamycin is a VERY safe drug. However, rapamycin initially developed a negative reputation because it was originally classified as an immunosuppressant to prevent organ rejection in patients who had received a kidney transplant. Suppressing the immune system is not a characteristic that is associated with drugs or nutrients that increase lifespan.

When rapamycin is given daily to organ transplant patients, a rare side effect called starvation pseudo-diabetes (SPD) occasionally develops. However, this condition does not occur when rapamycin is given once weekly. At higher doses, it also occasionally causes painful mouth ulcers.

One consequence of rapamycin therapy that has been discussed in the medical literature relates to muscle mass. mTOR regulates protein synthesis. Thus, rapamycin has the ability to hinder the building of new muscle mass. Here's what is known at this time. There are two slightly different forms of mTOR: mTORC1 (complex 1) and mTORC2 (complex

2). In studies with mice, it appears that long-term activation of mTORC1 stimulates muscle damage and loss. However, inhibition of mTORC1 with rapamycin reportedly prevents age-related muscle loss.[155]

Rapamycin's effect on muscle mass certainly needs to be studied more. So far, this topic has only been studied in mice. We need to study this effect in humans, or at least in nonhuman primates. When rapamycin is taken once weekly, which is the protocol for life extension, rapamycin's inhibition of mTORC1 seems to prevent age-related muscle loss. I feel that rapamycin's benefits far outweigh any potential side effects, and overall, rapamycin use in animals and humans to date has a remarkably safe safety profile.

In the article titled **"Rapamycin for Longevity"**, Dr. Blagosklonny also stated that "rather than being classified as an immunosuppressant, it would have been better to classify rapamycin as an immunomodulator and an anti-inflammatory drug." He also stated that "at anti-aging doses, rapamycin eliminates hyper-immunity rather than suppresses immunity or, more figuratively, it rejuvenates immunity.[156]

Side Effects of Rapamycin vs Aspirin

At the normal doses used for life extension, rapamycin's side effects are not much more dangerous than aspirin. Aspirin is one of the most commonly used over-the-counter drugs in the world. However, occasionally, aspirin can cause episodes of gastric bleeding and if taken in very high doses, there are several potentially serious side effects. Nevertheless, millions of people take aspirin regularly as an analgesic, as a mild blood thinner, and to reduce risks of cardiovascular disease and cancer. Thus, most people believe that aspirin's benefits outweigh its risks. Much the same can be said for rapamycin: its health benefits and life extension capabilities are much greater than the low risk of side effects.

Can You Overdo mTOR Inhibition?

Yes. It is well established that high-dose rapamycin and extensive mTOR inhibition causes immunosup-

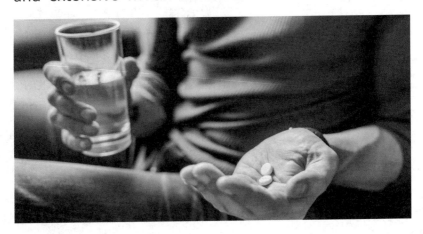

pression. That aspect is used beneficially to prevent organ rejection.

However, various other compounds and lifestyle factors are classified as mTOR inhibitors. Too much of a good thing can result in bad outcomes. Let's imagine an individual who is taking 6 mg of rapamycin once weekly. If this individual also decides to take metformin, engage in intermittent fasting and strength training and take one or more of the nutritional mTOR inhibitors (discussed in Chapter 12), one could begin to develop some side effects such as excessive loss of body fat, muscle, and/or bone density. The bottom line is to avoid overusing rapamycin and excessively inhibiting mTOR.

> "Too much of a good thing can result in bad outcomes. The bottom line is to avoid overuse of rapamycin and/or excessive inhibition of mTOR."

What's more, a few people who take rapamycin report developing canker sores (also called aphthous ulcers). These small, shallow lesions—which occur more frequently in people taking rapamycin daily or at higher doses—develop on the soft tissue inside your mouth or at the base of your gums. While not contagious, they can be painful. Fortunately, they are usually transient and resolve relatively quickly.

How to Track Your Rapamycin Progress

As previously mentioned, rapamycin given at lower doses and once weekly vs daily dosing has been shown to be remarkably safe. However, no long-term human trials have been conducted yet. The main metrics to track are the following:

a. How do you feel?

b. How is your overall energy?

c. Be mindful of your body weight. People who are overweight or obese will want to lose weight. However, rapid weight loss or losing too much weight could be a sign of rapamycin toxicity or over-inhibition of mTOR.

d. Keep tabs on your blood sugar. Taking too much rapamycin, or too much mTOR inhibition, can cause hypoglycemia. This ties in with item (b) which is your overall energy.

e. Don't obsess over your triglycerides. Studies on rapamycin's effect on serum triglycerides are conflicting and confusing. Some studies in mice report that rapamycin causes elevated triglycerides. Others report lower triglycerides. One meta-analysis of human trials concluded that kidney transplant patients taking high rapamycin doses on a daily basis had higher triglyceride and cholesterol levels. Health-promoting once-weekly dosing of rapamycin likely won't have this effect.

f. Track your serum iron and hemoglobin levels, but not too closely. Since mTOR is involved in the control of iron metabolism, it's thought that inhibiting its activity with rapamycin could inhibit iron accumulation and lead to low iron levels. Again, this is typically seen in patients taking rapamycin every day, not once per week.

My recommendation: I strongly encourage you to get a comprehensive panel of laboratory tests so you have a baseline reading of your triglycerides, cholesterol, iron, and hemoglobin levels. This will enable you to compare your baseline values with follow-up labs after you have been taking rapamycin for a while.

CHAPTER TEN

How to Get Your Rapamycin Prescription Filled and Covered by Insurance.

Dosage and Directions.

Rapamycin, which was assigned the generic name sirolimus, is a prescription drug that is distributed by Wyeth Pharmaceutical, which is a subsidiary of Pfizer, Inc. The brand name for rapamycin is Rapamune.

Sirolimus (aka rapamycin) is available in the following strengths:

- 0.5 mg tan triangular-shaped tablet
- 1.0 mg white triangular-shaped tablet
- 2.0 mg yellowish-beige triangular tablet
- 1 g/ml oral solution

At What Age Can People Start Taking Rapamycin?

No studies have evaluated this yet. However, it is well established that rapamycin and other mTOR inhibitors reduce cellular signals that regulate growth. In the human life cycle, childhood and adolescence are periods of rapid growth, hence it is probably inappropriate to give rapamycin to children or teenagers. Several of the rapamycin scientists I interviewed suggested that people younger than 25 years old should not take rapamycin. However, the incidence of metabolic syndrome and obesity, which are signs of mTOR Syndrome, are skyrocketing. Thus, decisions regarding who, and at what age, people should be prescribed rapamycin are decisions that physicians will need to make on an individualized basis.

How to Get Your Doctor to Write You a Prescription for Rapamycin

NOTE: These days, many physicians work in large group practices, which have strict rules and "standard of care" guidelines that they are required to follow. Thus, physicians in large group medical practices may be unwilling to write a prescription for rapamycin, which is a drug they are not familiar with and that is also outside their standard of care practice guidelines. You will have a much better chance of getting your doctor to write a prescription for rapamycin if you have developed a personal relationship with him/her.

Finding a physician who is willing to write a prescription for rapamycin will be difficult for many people. However, there is hope. As the life extension benefits of rapamycin begin to be more widely publicized, I think more physicians will want to begin taking it themselves. Also, since most physicians really are concerned about the health and wellbeing of their patients, and since rapamycin's benefits are so profound, I think an increasing number of physicians will be willing to write rapamycin prescriptions for their patients. This is one of the primary goals of this book.

A not-for-profit group called the *Age Reversal Network* maintains a listing of physicians who are knowledgeable about rapamycin and more likely to prescribe it for anti-aging purposes. You can access their physician's referral list at: https://age-reversal. net/physician-directory/.

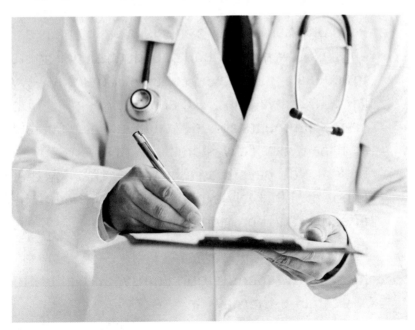

The *Age Reversal Network* may also make referrals to telehealth physicians who can assist people in obtaining rapamycin and other medications that have demonstrated anti-aging properties. I suggest you join the Age Reversal Network (www.age-reversal.net) at no cost so they can keep you updated about developments in the human longevity field.

I want to make the following suggestions, which I hope will help enlighten your existing physician. Before you ask your physician to write you a prescription for rapamycin, I suggest you do the following:

a. Become familiar with the materials discussed in this book and read, study, and/or listen to the educational materials provided in Chapter 8.

b. Read Dr. Thomas Levy's article in which he presents his viewpoints about a patient's legal rights to request and receive IV vitamin C therapy. Levy is both a physician (MD) and a lawyer (JD). Dr. Levy's comments about IV vitamin C also pertain to rapamycin. Levy states the following, "As a patient, you have the right to any therapy that is not prohibitively expensive, established to be effective, and not prohibitively toxic."

Link to Dr. Levy's article:

https://www.dcnutrition.com/your-rights-to-iv-vitamin-c-therapy/

or do an Internet search for *your rights to IV vitamin C therapy.*

c. Write a *"Statement of Personal Responsibility"* and provide it to your physician. This statement should simply state that you understand the risks and take full responsibility for your decision to take rapamycin.

Most physicians will not be familiar with rapamycin. Thus, you will probably need to start by educating your doctor about rapamycin. The purpose of this book is to educate you AND your doctor about the benefits and safety of rapamycin. I suggest emphasizing the following points:

- Rapamycin is very safe; it has been used safely by millions of patients since it gained FDA approval in September 1999.

- Print out and give your doctor a copy the article titled Rapamycin for longevity: opinion article, written by Dr. Mikhail Blagosklonny), or send him/her the link to the article (do an Internet search for *"Rapamycin for longevity: opinion article"*). It is an excellent review that explains how and why rapamycin functions as a life extension drug (Internet hyperlink is provided in Part 8). In the article, Dr. Blagosklonny makes the following statement:

"I will also discuss why it is more dangerous not to use anti-aging drugs than to use them and how rapamycin-based drug combinations have already been implemented for potential life extension in humans. *If you read this article from the very beginning to its end, you may realize that the time is now."*

- Encourage your doctor to listen to one or more of the following podcast interviews (links in Chapter 12).

  a. Peter Attia's interview with Dr. David Sabatini. Dr. Sabatini is the discoverer of mTOR; rapamycin's ability to inhibit mTOR is central to understanding the how rapamycin promotes health and life extension.

  b. Peter Attia's interview with Joan Mannick & Nir Barzilai

  c. Tim Ferriss' interview with Peter Attia.

- If your doctor refuses to write you a prescription for rapamycin, then you may want to consider finding another doctor.

Where and How to Get Your Rapamycin Rx Filled

MY STORY: Rapamycin is a fairly expensive drug. The average wholesale price (AWP) for a bottle of #100 rapamycin 2 mg tablets is $3,149.73. This is the price a pharmacy must pay when ordering rapamycin from their local drug wholesaler.

I initially took my rapamycin prescription to my local independent pharmacy, Ashland Drug, which is located in my hometown of Ashland, Oregon. After looking rapamycin up in the computer, the pharmacist/owner said, "It's available, but I won't fill it for you." Because my prescription is for only 12 tablets per month, the pharmacist explained that rapamycin is too expensive to have that much of their inventory tied up and sitting on his shelf.

I then took my rapamycin prescription to the local Rite Aid pharmacy. Rite Aid ordered the rapamycin and two days later I picked up my prescription. My point in explaining this is to let you know that chain drug stores are more likely to be willing to order rapamycin and fill your prescription whereas independent retail pharmacies may decline because it ties up too much money.

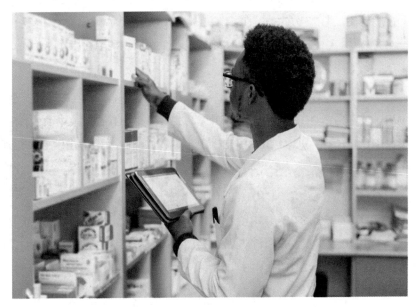

Insurance Coverage for Rapamycin

Insurance Companies: There are many different insurance programs. I will only comment on mine. When my pharmacist filled my rapamycin prescription, my BlueCross/BlueShield copay was $20. Insurance companies nowadays are seeking to deny payment for expensive medications. I discuss lower cost rapamycin sources a bit later in this book.

Medicare: According to GoodRx. All Medicare prescription drug plans cover rapamycin/sirolimus. https://www.goodrx.com/sirolimus/medicare-coverage. However, getting a prescription covered on Medicare requires that you have Medicare Part D coverage (D = coverage for drugs). Medicare prescription coverage also requires that the prescribing physician provide a diagnostic code, which denotes which illness is being treated. There are no codes for health and aging.

Compounding Pharmacies: I fear many readers will not be able to find affordable sources of name brand rapamycin because of its outlandish price.

The encouraging news is that more compounding pharmacies are making it 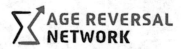 available in strengths not available by name brand companies, such as 5.5–6.5 mg once-per-week dosing. The Age Reversal Network—the not-for-profit group mentioned earlier—seeks to keep its members informed about compounding pharmacies offering low-cost rapamycin. I suggest you join the Age Reversal Network by logging on to www.age-reversal.net.

Recommended Dosage & Direction

First, I want to emphasize that large scale clinical trials to evaluate and determine the best dosage and directions for humans use of rapamycin and/or rapalogs have not been conducted yet. However, the human clinical trial conducted by Joan Mannick, MD did provide some important guidelines.

Dr. Joan Mannick Landmark Human Clinical Trial

In 2010, Dr. Joan Mannick was a senior scientist at Novartis and her passion was conducting research on the biology of aging. Dr. Mannick devised a human clinical trial using the drug RAD001 (also known as everolimus), which is a rapalog with effects very similar to rapamycin.[108] The 218 subjects selected for this trial were elderly people who were over 65 years of age. Most people of this age have experienced a significant decline in the function of their immune system compared to younger individuals.

In this trial, all subjects took rapamycin or placebo for six weeks. The subjects for this trial were divided into the following three groups:

1. Subjects received 0.5 mg of RADOO1 daily for 6 weeks or a placebo
2. Subjects received 5.0 mg of RADOO1 once weekly for 6 weeks or a placebo
3. Subjects received 20 mg of RADOO1 once weekly for 6 weeks of a placebo

Following the six week drug-phase, there was a 2-week drug-free wash out period. Then, all of the subjects were administered the seasonal flu vaccine.

After the flu vaccine was administered, the results revealed that the 5 mg dose taken once weekly proved to be the "sweet spot," resulting in about a 20% enhancement in immune system response to the flu vaccine.

The Mannick trial was important for two reasons. First, it was a human clinical trial which revealed that administration of rapamycin-like mTOR inhibitors could provide health benefits to elderly individuals. Second, this study documented that a moderate dose of rapamycin-like drugs taken once weekly provided superior benefits compared to either daily dosing or a high dose given once weekly.

Based on the information gleaned from the Mannick trial, the 5 mg dose of rapamycin taken once weekly is the dose that is most commonly prescribed by physicians for patients who are interested in life extension and healthy aging. This dosage regime is NOT based on a thorough survey of physicians who are prescribing and/or using rapamycin. It is simply the dose that virtually all of the physicians I spoke to in the process of writing this book admitted to using or prescribing.

RAPAMYCIN— NO PRESCRIPTION REQUIRED!

For people without insurance or if your doctor refuses to write a prescription for rapamycin, here's an excellent option. **International Antiaging Systems** (IAS) is a company that markets hard-to-obtain life extension products—including a generic brand of rapamycin called RapaPro (produced to ISO and cGMP standards). What's more, the rapamycin is nano-sized and the tablets are film-coated for enhanced bioavailability.

The price for 50 RapaPro 1 mg tablets is $69.99, which is the best price I have seen for rapamycin. Also, you can get a 10% discount on your first order by using code ROSS-10 at checkout. To learn more, visit www.Antiaging-Systems.com.

FDA Reform Urgently Needed: Get the FDA to Classify Aging as a Disease

The FDA views aging as a natural process. Consequently, they do not allow aging to be classified as a disease. This policy limits and obstructs the ability to study aging since companies have virtually no chance of getting the FDA to approve clinical trials to evaluate drugs, biologics, or other interventions that may slow or reverse biological aging processes.

Many health care professionals think the FDA is sadly out of date and drastically in need of modernization. Here are some examples of FDA overregulation that stifles human studies:

1. Currently available drugs that may slow aging are too expensive
2. Approval process too long and cumbersome
3. High cost of clinical trials creates quasi-monopoly for Big Pharma
4. Revolving door: FDA employees can leave to become high-paid consultants for companies they regulated.
5. Refusal to recognize aging as a disease

The way most clinical trials have sought FDA approval is to target specific degenerative disorders such as Alzheimer's, cardiovascular disease, diabetes, and sarcopenia—but not systemic aging itself.

I began advocating for FDA reform in 1989 when I wrote my first book, *Mind, Food, & Smart Pills*, which describes various nootropic drugs and nutrients. I wrote about drugs named piracetam and meclofenoxate (Lucidril), which are cognitive-enhancing drugs that improve cognitive function and slow down the progression of brain aging.

Piracetam and meclofenoxate are relatively inexpensive drugs available in many countries throughout the world, but not in the United States. This makes me angry. I hope it makes you angry, too. Please speak up and make your voice heard. Contact your state and federal political representatives and request fast action on FDA reforms. And if you call or write, please be sure to emphasize your desire to have aging classified as a disease.

The goal of medicine should be to help people attain and maintain good health for as long as possible. If the FDA would change its policy and allow aging to be classified as a disease, it would dramatically increase funding for aging research and the development of products that slow down the process of biological aging.

There is a growing movement among scientists and life extension enthusiasts to convince the FDA that aging itself should be classified as a disease. This would encourage companies and the government to fund research on new drugs, products, and therapies that treat aging.

Currently, the annual budget for the National Institutes of Health (NIH) is about $45 billion. The National Institute on Aging (NIA), which is one of the 27 Institutes and Centers of NIH, has an annual budget of about $4 billion. Over 90% of NIH's budget is devoted to research on individual diseases, and less than 10% is devoted to aging research through the NIA.

But if you take a close look at the NIA's website, you'll find that much of their funding is devoted to supporting and conducting Alzheimer's disease research. This means that very little money is devoted to researching the fundamental process of aging.

If, like me, you'd like this to change, please become politically active. Call your political representatives and urge them to get the FDA to classify aging as a disease.

To sign a petition asking the FDA to allow aging Americans to "opt out" of today's rigid clinical-trials mandate so they can experiment with interventions that might extend healthy human life, log on to www.age-reversal.net/FDA.

Proposed Medical Freedom Amendment

In that same vein, the National Health Federation board member Michael LeVesque has proposed a long awaited Twenty-Eighth Amendment—the Medical Freedom Amendment—to the US Constitution's Bill of Rights, which would protect an individual's right to medical privacy and choice. The amendment states the following:

"All people have the Right to secure their Health in the manner they choose. Congress, the President, State Legislatures and Executives, Governmental Agencies or Departments shall make no law or executive order that impedes the Individual's rights to informed consent nor right to medical choice nor freedom of medical choice. Nor shall the President, Congress, State Legislatures, and Executives, Governmental Agencies, or Departments make any law or executive order that impedes the Individual's right to medical privacy and freedom without individual and specific judicial warrant supported by Oath and affirmation of necessary cause to protect Society from Harm describing the Individual's condition and danger it presents."

For more information, or to join this movement, go to: http://medicalfreedomamendment.org/

CHAPTER ELEVEN

Summarizing the Importance of Rapamycin, mTOR, and Autophagy

I believe the Rapamycin/mTOR/Autophagy story is one of the most important discoveries in the history of mankind. In chapter three, I mentioned that Yoshinori Ohsumi was awarded the 2016 Nobel Prize in physiology and medicine for discovering the mechanism of autophagy. I would not be surprised if a Nobel Prize was awarded at some future date to the scientists who discovered mTOR.

Early studies suggested that rapamycin had anticancer activity. Studies at the U.S. National Cancer Institute (NCI) not only confirmed this, but also reported that rapamycin may be a totally different kind of cancer drug that would be produce far fewer side effects than traditional cytotoxic cancer drugs. These exciting reports stimulated surge in rapamycin research based on the desire to understand rapamycin's mechanism, i.e. how, exactly, does rapamycin work?

In some cancer studies, rapamycin has not been as effective as anticipated. However, additional studies have reported that rapamycin used in conjunction with another chemotherapy protocol might enhance overall outcomes.[158]

In 1994, David Sabatini, Stuart Schreiber and Robert Abraham independently discovered rapamycin binds to an enzyme protein within cells that was named mTOR, which stands for *mechanistic target of rapamycin*. Now, 28 years after its discovery, over 11,000 papers have been published on mTOR. It is now well understood that mTOR is a central regulator of cellular processes that influence lifespan and aging.

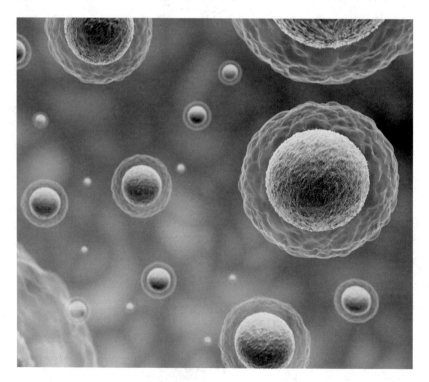

Now we understand that mTOR functions like the gas pedal that regulates cellular metabolism and cellular growth processes. On the other hand, inhibiting mTOR (like rapamycin does) functions like the brake pedal, putting growth processes into a resting mode. This allows autophagy to then begin the processes of removal of trash or cellular housekeeping, which is vital to repair and revitalization of cells throughout the body.

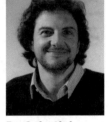

Dr. Sabatini

Regular periods of autophagy are critical for health and longevity. When autophagy is not engaged at regular intervals, cellular trash builds up, damaged proteins do not get replaced and recycled and the consequences are accelerated onset of diseases and accelerated aging.

An Epidemic of Epidemics

Although infectious diseases in developed economies have largely been eliminated, mankind is now experiencing an epidemic of chronic degenerative diseases.[159]

We suffer from an epidemic of cancer[160], cardiovascular disease[161], inflammatory bowel diseases[162], metabolic syndrome[163], obesity[164], arthritis[165], Alzheimer's disease[166], autism[167], ADHD[168], nonalcoholic fatty liver disease (NAFLD)[169], depression, anxiety and other forms of mental illness.[170] It is unprecedented to have so many types of chronic degenerative diseases escalating to epidemic proportions all at the same time. Mankind is experiencing an epidemic of epidemics.

One of the most important keys to understanding, and hopefully reversing, mankind's declining health, especially as it relates to obesity and a host of related disorders, is to educate people about mTOR and autophagy. Both processes are a necessary part of life. The health problems I mentioned are due to the fact that mTOR and autophagy are severely out of balance. I previously mentioned that our ancient ancestors probably spent twice as much time in the autophagy state compared to modern humans.

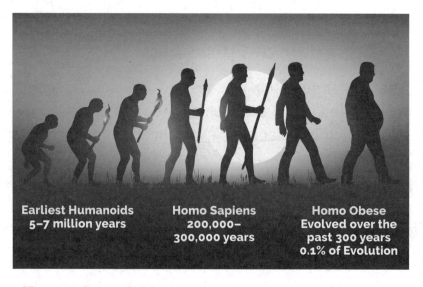

Earliest Humanoids
5–7 million years

Homo Sapiens
200,000–
300,000 years

Homo Obese
Evolved over the
past 300 years
0.1% of Evolution

There are a number of factors that have contributed to the decline in time spent in autophagy, such as refrigeration and the easy availability of food in grocery stores and convenience stores. The net result is that people spend far too much time consuming food and not enough time in periods of fasting.

The Timing of When You Eat

Health problems such as obesity, metabolic syndrome, and type 2 diabetes are major problems. However, the primary way that people try to correct these problems is by either eating less (how much they eat) and/or changing their diets (what they eat). The importance of the timing of when people eat has largely been neglected in the thinking of most people.

As mentioned earlier, for most of mankind's evolution, people did not eat breakfast, lunch, and dinner, interspersed with between-meal and bedtime snacks. I know I'm repeating myself, but this topic is critical to understanding long-term health, and why rapamycin works so well. Our ancestors, who ate 1 or 2 meals a day, only spent about 4 hours consuming food daily. Many people today are eating from 7 AM until 9 PM, which means they are consuming calories 14-hours per day compared to our ancestors who consumed calories 4-hours/day. Consequently, mTOR is activated for much longer each day and the critical process of autophagy doesn't seldom gets activated, which has devastating health consequences.

Research into rapamycin's mechanisms of action have elucidated the importance of autophagy, and its relative absence in the lives of most people.

Calorie restriction and intermittent fasting are very important, but most people won't adhere to these protocols. This is what rapamycin does for you; by mimicking calorie restriction, it initiates autophagy without you having to engage in calorie restriction or fasting. In the future, I hope someone conducts a rapamycin study comparing people who eat 3 meals a day vs people who are engaged in intermittent fasting. I'd bet that combining rapamycin with intermittent fasting will increase the positive results.

Refer to Chapter 5 for the discussion of calorie restriction and intermittent fasting.

CHAPTER TWELVE

The Science:
Links to Key Scientific Studies, Articles, and Podcast Interviews

I've read, listened to, and studied literally hundreds of studies, articles and podcast interviews on rapamycin over the past two years. In this chapter, I provide some links to mTOR and autophagy because these topics are intimately linked to understanding rapamycin's benefits. I've compiled what I consider to be the best resources to accelerate the rapamycin learning curve for you and your physician.

PODCASTS & INTERVIEWS

- **Peter Attia, MD interviews Dr. David Sabatini, MD, PhD** in episode #90 on Attia's podcast named *The Drive*. Sabatini is credited with discovering the mTOR signaling pathway, which explains the health benefits associated with rapamycin. Do an Internet search for the names **"Attia Sabatini"** or use the following link: https://peterattiamd.com/davidsabatini/

- **Joe Rogan interviews Dr. Peter Attia** in episode #1108 on his podcast, *The Joe Rogan Experience*. Joe is an excellent interviewer and Peter Attia articulately explains how rapamycin works and how important it is for health and longevity. Do an Internet search for the names **"Rogan Attia"** or use the following link: https://open.spotify.com/episode/1rVmRJzW9wqnZrYDJlRu42

- **Peter Attia, MD interviews Joan Mannick, MD & Nir Barzilai, MD** on episode #123 of *The Drive*. Topics covered are Rapamycin and Metformin—Longevity, Immune Enhancement and COVID-19. Do an Internet search for the terms **"Attia Mannick"** or use the following link:

  https://peterattiamd.com/joanmannick-nirbarzilai/

- **Peter Attia, MD interviews Lloyd Klickstein, MD, PhD** on episode #118 of *The Drive*. In this interview Dr. Klickstein discusses rapamycin, mTOR inhibition and the biology of aging. Do an Internet search for the terms **"Attia Klickstein"** or use the following link: https://peterattiamd.com/lloydklickstein/

- **Tim Ferriss' interview with Peter Attia** on episode #517 of *The Tim Ferriss Show*. Topics discussed are Longevity Drugs, Alzheimer's Disease, and the 3 Most Important Levers to

Pull. Do an Internet search for **"Ferriss Attia"** or use the following link: https://tim.blog/2021/06/08/peter-attia-2/

- **Radiolab Podcast : May 21, 2021.** *The Dirty Drug and the Ice Cream Tub*. This episode of Radiolab recounts the amazing journey of rapamycin, from its initial discovery on Easter Island to how it was almost discarded, and how samples of rapamycin were illegally smuggled from Canada into the United States. This eventually led to studies that ultimately revealed that rapamycin might be the most important life extension drug yet discovered. Part of the rapamycin story is told through the lens of the wife and son of Suren Sehgal, who is the scientist who originally discovered rapamycin in the soil samples taken years earlier from Easter Island. This episode also contains comments from David Sabatini and Matt Kaeberlein, who have also played important roles in the rapamycin story.

  Here is the link to this podcast: https://www.wnycstudios.org/podcasts/radiolab/articles/dirty-drug-and-ice-cream-tub

  Or do an Internet search for the terms: **"Radiolab May 2021 Rapamycin"**.

SCIENTIFIC STUDIES & ARTICLES

- **"Rapamycin for Longevity: Opinion Article"** by Mikhail Blagosklonny, which was published in the Oct. 15, 2019 issue of the journal *Aging*;11(19): pages 8048–67. Dr. Blagosklonny's article is the best summary of the history and science of rapamycin and its importance as a life-extension drug. To read this article, just to an Internet search for *"Rapamycin for Longevity: Opinion Article."*

- **"Cellular Housekeeping"** by William Faloon who is co-founder of the Life Extension group. This article was published in the March 2021 issue of the *Life Extension* magazine. To access this article, do an Internet search for: Life Extension Magazine March 2021. Then click on Download Magazine PDF (pages 7–11).

I joined Life Extension group when it was founded in 1980 by William Faloon and Saul Kent. I have been a member of the Life Extension's Medical Advisory Board for over 20 years, and I consider the monthly *Life Extension* magazine to be one of my most important sources of cutting-edge information about life extension products, science, and technology.

The Life Extension group has extremely high standards for quality control and the quality of the ingredients in their nutritional formulas.

One of their products is called "AMPK Metabolic Activator" and it contains ingredients that indirectly suppress excess mTOR.

Another called "Autophagy Renew" contains ingredients shown to promote autophagy. For those who have difficulty obtaining rapamycin, these modestly priced nutritional formulas can be ordered at **www. LifeExtension.com/TOR**.

To stay current with new data on suppressing mTOR and inducing autophagy, I encourage readers to obtain a free Life Extension Magazine subscription by logging on to **www.LifeExtension.com/TOR**.

- **"Rapamycin: One drug, many effects"** was published in the March 4, 2014 issue of *Cellular Metabolism* (authors Li, Kim and Blenis). To read this article do an Internet search for *"Rapamycin: One drug, many effects"*.

- **"Effect of rapamycin on aging and age-related diseases—past and future"** which was published in the Oct. 10, 2020 issue of the journal *GeroScience* (authors Selvarani, Mohammed and Richardson). To read this article, just to an Internet search for the title of the article.

- **"Rapamycin: Prevention & Treatment of Aging and Age-Related Disease"** by Alan S. Green, MD. This article is posted on Dr. Green's website which is: https://rapamycintherapy.com/

- **"mTOR as Regulator of Lifespan, Aging and Cellular Senescence: A Mini-Review",** which was published in the 2018 issue of the journal *Gerontology* (64(2):127–34). To read this article, do an Internet search for the title of the article.

VIDEOS

- In 2016, CNN aired a video showing a 13-year-old dog named Mono who races around the yard like a puppy after being on rapamycin for only 6 months. To view this short video, do an Internet search for the terms: "CNN dog rapamycin" (a 30-second ad runs before the dog video starts).

- 3-minute video introducing the PEARL trial, which is the first clinical trial designed to test rapamycin for healthy life extension in humans. To view this video, do an Internet search for the following terms: **"rapamycin pearl video"** or use the following link: https://www.lifespan.io/campaigns/pearl-participatory-evaluation-of-aging-with-rapamycin-for-longevity/

CHAPTER THIRTEEN

Alan Green, MD:
Utilizing Rapamycin in the Prevention and Treatment of Aging and Age-Related Diseases in Over 1,200 Patients

This chapter is a profile of Alan Green, MD, who is a board-certified pathologist. Dr. Green has transformed his practice; he now specializes in the treatment of age-related diseases, and he currently has over 1,200 patients taking rapamycin.

Several years ago, Dr. Green had some personal health problems that he was increasingly worried about. During 2014 and 2015, his energy level and his cardiovascular function were rapidly declining, and he thought that he probably only had 2 or 3 years left to live. In 2016, Dr. Green read Mikhail Blagosklonny's article titled **Rapamycin for Longevity** (referenced in Part 8: Articles)[122]. The article explained how rapamycin works and summarized the many benefits including life extension that had been reported from rapamycin studies. The data was compelling, so Dr. Green elected to start taking rapamycin in January 2016. Within 3 months of starting rapamycin, Dr.

Green said he felt 5 to 10 years younger. His cardio-vascular function and his energy levels had greatly improved. Based on his own dramatic improvements, Dr. Green started prescribing rapamycin to his patients in April 2017.

> Within 3 months of starting rapamycin, Dr. Green said he felt 5 to 10 years younger. His cardiovascular function and his energy levels had greatly improved.

Dr. Green's story is an excellent example of a physician who learned about rapamycin, understood its importance and safety, started taking it himself, experienced significant health improvements personally...and then began recommending it and prescribing it for his patients.

I conducted a personal interview with Dr. Green on July 18, 2021. During our discussion, he disclosed that he has prescribed rapamycin to over 700 patients.

On his website, Dr. Green makes the following statement, **"Rapamycin is the most important new drug since the 1928 discovery of penicillin and the dawn of antibiotics."** The heading at the top of Dr. Green's website states: **Rapamycin: Prevention & Treatment of Aging and Age-Related Diseases.**

The website for Dr. Green's medical practice is: **www.rapamycintherapy.com**.

His website contains a detailed discussion of his use of rapamycin in his patients along with information about other drugs and nutrients with known benefits for life extension.

CHAPTER FOURTEEN

Non-Prescription Indirect mTOR Inhibitors/ AMPK Activators

AMPK is an enzyme within all cells that can activate autophagy in a pathway that differs from mTOR inhibition. Hence, products that activate AMPK represent another category of compounds that promote autophagy and cellular regenerative processes.

AMPK is another evolutionarily conserved mechanism that has been regulating cellular metabolism for millennia, long before plants, animals and humans began to evolve.

AMPK acts as an energy sensor within cells. It is activated when cellular energy levels (ATP) are low, which initiates cellular autophagy. AMPK activators are being increasingly recognized as an important new class of anti-aging compounds.

For people who have difficulty convincing a physician to prescribe them rapamycin, natural AMPK activators offer reasonably priced alternative solutions to inhibiting mTOR and increasing autophagy.

Here are some natural AMPK inhibitors that promote autophagy.

1. **Intermittent fasting** (already discussed)

2. **Caloric restriction** (already discussed)

3. **Exercise** "uses up" energy. When nutrients and cellular energy are in short supply, AMPK is activated, which in turn promotes autophagy. Both moderate and high intensity exercise have been shown to activate AMPK. Exercise-induced activation of AMPK and subsequent activation of autophagy is one reason why regular exercise is critical to health and healthy aging.[172]

4. **Luteolin** is flavonoid compound that is found in vegetables and fruits such as celery, parsley, broccoli, onion leaves, carrots, peppers, cabbages, and apple skins. Studies have reported that luteolin activates autophagy and improves cellular metabolism.[173] Other reported beneficial effects of luteolin include the following: antioxidant, anti-inflammatory, neuroprotection, and improvement in memory.[174]

5. **Piperlongumine** is a spice that occurs in the long pepper plant (also called the Indian long pepper), which is a native to India. Piperlongumine has been shown to activate AMPK (which indirectly inhibits mTOR) and numerous publications have reported on its anti-cancer activity.[174]

Recall that rapamycin directly suppresses mTOR and induces beneficial autophagy. For those challenged to obtain affordable rapamycin, a nutritional formula called "Autophagy Renew" contains precise doses of luteolin and piperlongumine in one daily capsule. This formula can be ordered at **LifeExtension.com/TOR**.

6. **Curcumin** is a bright yellow compound that is the active ingredient in the turmeric plant. It is used widely as a dietary spice and in herbal medicine. Curcumin has many well-documented health benefits which include increasing lifespan, promoting weight loss, and reducing risks to heart disease, inflammation, neurodegenerative disease, cancer and depression.[176]

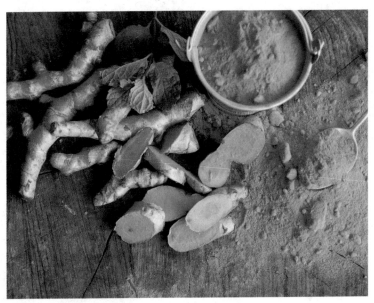

Curcumin has been shown to induce autophagy by activating the AMPK signaling pathway.[177] In animal studies (nematode, fruit flies and mice), curcumin has been shown to increase mean lifespan.[178]

Poor absorption and low bioavailability have limited the therapeutic effectiveness of curcumin because it gets quickly metabolized into inactive forms and is eliminated from the body.[179] A novel patented technology that combines curcumin with specific type of fiber derived from fenugreek seeds has been shown to dramatically increase the absorption of curcumin. Results from absorption studies with this new formula reported an astounding 45.5-fold increase in the bioavailability of curcumin compared to standard curcumin formulations.[180] High bioavailable curcumin products using this new patented formulation are available from Life Extension at LifeExtension.com/rapa.

7. **Gynostemma pentaphyllum** is a Chinese herbal plant that is distantly related to the cucumber. It is widely used in Asia as to treat obesity, type 2 diabetes, elevated blood lipids, and inflammation.[181] Asian doctors recommend G. pentaphyllum to promote longevity. Recent studies report that some of G. pentaphyllum's health benefits are

due to its ability to activate the AMPK signaling pathway.[182] A Life Extension product named AMPK Metabolic Activator contains Actiponin, which is a patented brand of *Gynostemma* extract.

8. **Green tea (Camellia sinensis)** has been used for its medicinal properties in Asian cultures for thousands of years. One of the main compounds in green tea, named epigallocatechin gallate (EGCG) has recently been found to activate AMPK activity and promote autophagy.[183] This may help explain some of the many health benefits attributed to green tea.

CHAPTER FIFTEEN

Metformin: A True Anti-Aging Drug?

Metformin is an FDA-approved drug that has been used successfully for over 60 years to treat diabetes.

In fact, metformin is the most commonly prescribed drug in the world for the treatment of type 2 diabetes.

Because metformin effectively lowers both blood glucose and blood insulin levels[184], it also reduces the risk to many other chronic degenerative diseases[185].

Consequently, in addition to its use in the treatment of type 2 diabetes, metformin is now being tested as a therapy to slow down aging. In January 2017, I posted

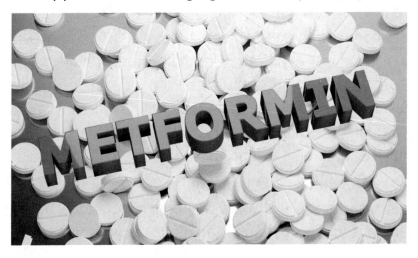

an article on my blog titled *Metformin: A True Anti-Aging Drug* (available at **www.naturalpharmacist.net**).

In 2016 the FDA made an unprecedented announcement when it approved a study to examine the effect of metformin on the biology of aging in humans. This study is titled *Targeting Aging with Metformin*, or the *TAME* study. This is the first time in history that the FDA has approved any human clinical trial with a goal of establishing a drug's ability to protect against multiple diseases of aging.

In previous studies in worms, flies, mice and rats, administration of metformin has resulted in significant increases in lifespan. Many healthy people are now electing to take metformin for its ability to slow down aging processes and increase longevity.

Metformin: An AMPK Activator

AMPK is a nutrient sensing enzyme that is present in all mammalian cells. In some ways, AMPK and mTOR are similar in that they both monitor energy and nutrient availability in cells. When cellular energy levels are low, AMPK activates signaling pathways that replenish cellular energy supplies, such as glucose uptake, fatty acid oxidation, and autophagy.[186]

Metformin works by inhibiting the synthesis of glucose in the liver, which in turn activates AMPK and autophagy. By inhibiting glucose synthesis in the liver, metformin enables the pancreas to reduce the production of insulin which results in lower levels of blood glucose and insulin[187]. This also results in an increase in insulin sensitivity, which means the cells' insulin receptors function better. Metformin also decreases appetite and food consumption, induces weight and fat loss, and decreases triglycerides and LDL-cholesterol levels.

Metformin's Anti-Cancer Benefits

The first study to explore metformin's anticancer benefits was conducted on hamsters in 2001. In this study, hamsters were divided into two groups, placed on a high-fat diet, and administered a chemical known to cause pancreatic cancer. One group received metformin in their drinking water and the other group received nothing and served as controls. At the end of 42 weeks, 50% of the hamsters in the high-fat group developed malignant tumors; however, none of the hamsters taking metformin developed tumors.[188]

In 2009, the results of a large metformin trial were published. In this 10-year trial, evaluating over 8,000 diabetic patients, it was discovered that diabetic patients taking metformin had a 54% lower risk of developing any type of cancer compared to diabetic patients who had not taken metformin. And, for people with cancer, metformin users had a much greater length of survival.[189]

Metformin & Obesity

Over two-thirds of Americans are either overweight or obese, and the health risks associated with being overweight are enormous.[190] The link between obesity and diabetes is so strong, these co-morbidities have given rise to the term 'diabesity'. In addition to improving control of blood glucose and blood insulin levels, studies have shown that metformin acts on the hypothalamus, resulting in a reduction in both food intake and body weight.[191,192]

The patent for metformin (brand name Gluco-phage) has expired, so metformin is now a very inexpensive generic drug. Taking metformin will help most adults regulate their blood glucose and insulin levels, which in turn will improve their long-term health and promote healthy longevity.

CHAPTER SIXTEEN

Can Rapamycin Reverse Aging?

In addition to extending lifespan in many species of animals, results from an increasing number of animal studies are reporting that rapamycin therapy can reverse some of the biomarkers of aging in some age-related diseases.

Below are summaries of some of these studies.

Study #1: mTOR Regulation and Therapeutic Rejuvenation of Aging Hematopoietic Stem Cells.[193]

Discussion: Hematopoietic stem cells (HSCs) are stem cells that are produced in the bone marrow, and they play important roles in regulation of the immune system. The activity of HSCs in young mice (2-months old) was found to be far greater than the HSCs from old (24-month-old) mice, which means the immune system of the old mice had declined substantially with age.

HSCs in old mice have elevated mTOR signaling.[194] In this study, scientists tried to determine whether treatment with rapamycin and subsequent inhibition of mTOR would reverse the decline in the function of the

HSCs and the decline in immune function of old mice. To test this hypothesis, the researchers divided 26-month-old mice into two groups. One group was treated with rapamycin for 6 weeks and the other group served as controls. After a 2-week wash-out period, all mice were injected with influenza virus. The mice that were pre-treated with rapamycin exhibited a much stronger immune response to the viral challenge.

This study revealed that treatment with rapamycin reversed the decline in the functional capacity of HSCs, and the age-related decline in the function of the immune system in aged mice. In another test to determine how effectively rapamycin treatment affected the response to vaccination in old mice, the mice were administered a dose of influenza virus that would normally be lethal to non-immunized young mice. Whereas 75% of the placebo-control mice died from the lethal dose of the virus, 100% of the rapamycin-treated mice survived.

Study #2: A randomized controlled trial to establish the effects of short-term rapamycin treatment in 24 middle-aged companion dogs.[195]

Discussion: Companion dogs (i.e. pets) share the same environment with their owners, are subject to similar risk factors, receive comparable medical care, and develop many of the same age-related diseases humans do.

Both humans and dogs experience a gradual decline in the functional capacity of the heart and immune system as they age. These declines are a hallmark of aging. In this study, 24 middle-aged dogs were administered either a placebo or rapamycin 3 times/week for 10 weeks. The dogs receiving rapamycin exhibited reversal of the age-related decline in several measures of cardiac function. A larger trial with 375 companion dogs is currently in progress; it is designed to validate rapamycin's effects on cardiac function and to determine if it can significantly improve healthspan and reduce mortality in companion dogs.

Study #3: Altered proteome turnover and remodeling by short-term caloric restriction or rapamycin rejuvenate the aging heart.[196]

Discussion: Two hallmarks of aging in the cardiovascular system are cardiac hypertrophy (an abnormal enlargement or thickening of the heart muscle) and diastolic dysfunction (a stiffening or inflexibility of the heart muscle that prevents the heart ventricles from filling completely).

This trial was designed to investigate the effect of two, short-term (10-week) therapeutic options, rapamycin or caloric restriction, on cardiac function in aging mice. The researchers examined a wide range of factors associated with cardiac function during aging. As expected, all of the markers deteriorated as the mice aged. However, in both the rapamycin-treated mice and the calorie-restricted mice, these markers were significantly reversed.

The authors of this study stressed that the results of this study demonstrate that instituting rapamycin therapy in old mice reverses many of the already developing functional deficits of cardiac aging, rather than just slowing down the aging process.

The Dog Aging Project: Enrolling 100,000 Dogs

The Dog Aging Project (DAP) is one of the largest long-term studies of aging ever conducted. The project, which was founded in 2014 at the University of Washington, has two primary goals: First, to understand how genes, lifestyle, and environmental factors influence aging. And second, to study interventions that can increase the healthspan and lifespan of dogs. The project plans to enroll tens of thousands of companion dogs (i.e., pets) and follow them for more than 10 years.

Why Study Dogs?

The fundamental long-term goal of the DAP is to study the biology of aging. Like humans, individual dogs vary in life expectancy and the spectrum of diseases they are likely to encounter. However, the biology and physiology of dogs is similar in many ways to humans. Dogs and humans have similar organ systems (heart, lungs, kidneys, liver, eyes, brain, etc.), have similar requirements for vitamins, minerals, and other nutrients, and make the same biological compounds such as cortisol, adrenaline, and dopamine.

Another benefit in studying dogs is that their age-related diseases are diagnosed and treated within a sophisticated veterinary healthcare system that parallels human healthcare in many ways.

Companion dogs age approximately 7 to 10 times faster than humans.

They also share the same physical and chemical environment as humans, a major determinant of aging that cannot be adequately modeled in laboratory studies. By studying the diseases of aging in dogs, the researchers hope to gain a better understanding of the factors that cause biological aging and identify potential interventions that can increase the healthspan and lifespan, not just in dogs but also in humans.

10-Week Rapamycin Trial

In 2017, the project reported results from a short 10-week trial with 24 middle-aged companion dogs, which revealed that dogs who had been treated with rapamycin had improvements in both systolic and diastolic cardiac function compared to placebo controls.[198] Based on these positive results and other preliminary studies, the DAP received a five-year grant from the National Institute on Aging (NIA) along with an additional $2.5 million from a group of tech entrepreneurs.

The Long-Term Dog Aging Project

The power of the DAP lies in its ability to capture the breadth of diversity of companion dogs and to collect a rich array of data about each dog. The greater the diversity, the greater the opportunity to characterize the age trajectory of diseases, to identify biomarkers, and to discover genetic and environmental risk factors for disease outcomes. The target study population consists of dogs of all breeds (both purebred and mixed breed), ages, sizes, and sexes (males and females, intact and sterilized).

Structurally, the DAP can be considered a collection of five overlapping cohorts, or groups, of dogs. The largest group of dogs is the "Pack," which consists of dogs whose owners successfully complete the Health and Life Experience Survey (HLES). Once enrolled, these dogs are members of the Pack for the dog's lifetime.

Following submission of a qualifying electronic veterinary medical record, dogs in the Pack become eligible for the other, more deeply studied cohorts in which owners are sent kits for biospecimen collection. The sampled cohorts include Foundation, Precision, Brain Health, and TRIAD (Test of Rapamycin In Aging Dogs), as well as a cross-sectional sample of extremely old "centenarian" dogs.

The Pack: The Pack consists of tens of thousands of dogs that will be followed for the entirety of their lives, utilizing regular surveys completed by the owners.

The Foundation: The aim of the Foundation cohort study is to provide a foundation (hence the name) of genetic information about a wide range of dogs. The DAP has grant funding to pay for low-pass sequencing of 10,000 dogs. Genome sequence data for canine participants will be integrated with health measures and behavioral traits to carry out comprehensive genome-wide association studies.

The Precision: This study takes a more precise look at how canine biology and physiology are related to aging. Participants in this cohort will utilize a DNA kit similar to that of the Foundation cohort members. After returning the saliva sample, the next step will be to request a sample kit to collect biological samples. Precision cohort members will need to take their dogs to their primary care veterinarians annually for the collection of these samples. In addition, owners of dogs in the Precision cohort will be asked to do other activities such as playing cognitive games with their dogs, taking body-size measurements, and timing their dogs during mobility assessments.

Brain Health Study: This study is funded by a second large NIH grant to specifically identify genetic and environmental factors that influence the risk of cognitive decline and dementia in companion dogs, a disorder called canine cognitive dysfunction. Up to 200 dogs with cognitive impairment or dementia will be sampled similarly to the Precision cohort.

The TRIAD: TRIAD stands for Test of Rapamycin in Aging Dogs. The TRIAD's goal is to conduct a double-blind, placebo-controlled clinical trial of the drug rapamycin. This cohort is smaller than either the Foundation or Precision cohorts, eventually enrolling 580 larger middle-aged dogs into the clinical trial. The eligibility process is much more involved and will take several months. Dogs included in the TRIAD must meet a series of specific eligibility requirements and attend a screening visit at a participating veterinary teaching hospital to ensure that they have no underlying health conditions that might prohibit their participation. Like Foundation and Precision members, those in the TRIAD eligibility process will receive DNA and sample kits.

Participation in the DAP is open to all geographical regions in the U.S. Participation is currently limited to one dog per household; however, there is no limit to the total number of dogs that can join the DAP's Pack. The DAP has four primary scientific aims, which include:

(1) Characterizing aging in companion dogs on three separate axes: multi-morbidity, frailty, and inflammaging.

(2) Using low-coverage whole-genome sequencing with imputation on at least 10,000 dogs to analyze the genetic architecture of age-related traits in dogs.

(3) Collecting metabolome, epigenome, and microbiome profiles to develop biomarkers of aging in dogs and to better understand the mechanisms by which genetic, environmental, and lifestyle variation influence aging.

(4) Carrying out a randomized, double-masked, placebo-controlled study to determine the effects of rapamycin on the onset and severity of age-related diseases.

Current Status

The DAP hopes to enroll 100,000 dogs in the Pack by the end of 2023. They are still enrolling dogs for the TRIAD/rapamycin trial. News and updates are available at: https://dogagingproject.org/

Meet the Dog Aging Project (DAP) Team

The DAP is headed by co-directors Matt Kaeberlein and Daniel Promislow, who are biologists and biogerontologists, and chief veterinarian, Dr. Kate Creevy. The DAP is an innovative study that brings together a community of dogs and their owners, veterinarians, scientists, and volunteers to carry out the most ambitious dog health study and the largest long-term study of biological aging in the world.

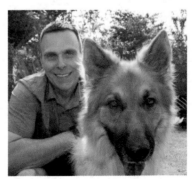

Matt Kaeberlein and his dog Dobby

Collaborating Institutions

Currently, there are 28 research organizations that are collaborating with the DAP. Collectively, these scientific organizations and institutions make a strong statement about the credibility and importance of the DAP for advancing our understanding of biological aging. What is learned from the DAP will eventually benefit the health and the lifespan of dogs—and humans.

- Arizona State University
- Broad Institute of MIT and Harvard
- Colorado State University Flint Animal Cancer Center
- Colorado State University College of Veterinary Medicine & Biomedical Sciences
- Cornell University College of Veterinary Medicine
- Fred Hutchinson Cancer Center
- Harvard Medical School Center for Bioethics
- Iowa State University College of Veterinary Medicine
- Midwestern University Animal Health Institute
- National University of Singapore
- North Carolina State College of Veterinary Medicine
- Oregon State University Carlson College of Veterinary Medicine
- Princeton University
- Seattle Children's Hospital
- Tel Aviv University
- Texas A&M University School of Veterinary Medicine & Biomedical Sciences
- University of Arizona
- University of Georgia College of Veterinary Medicine
- University of Massachusetts Chan Medical School
- University of Pennsylvania Center for Translational Bioinformatics
- University of Southern California
- University of Washington College of Arts & Sciences
- University of Washington College of Built Environments
- University of Washington School of Medicine
- University of Washington School of Public Health
- University of Wisconsin School of Medicine and Public Health
- Virginia-Maryland College of Veterinary Medicine, Virginia Tech
- Washington State University College of Veterinary Medicine

EPILOGUE

As researchers continue to explore the many health and longevity benefits rapamycin provides, its potential to extend both lifespan and healthspan can't be overstated. The goal of *Rapamycin, mTOR, Autophagy & Treating mTOR Syndrome* is to share these findings with practitioners and consumers. But this goal can't be accomplished without help. To that end, I'd like to share a profile of Dr. Steven Hotze, who is the founder and director of the Hotze Health & Wellness Center (HWC) located in Houston, Texas.

In June 2022, Dr. Don Ellsworth, one of the physicians at HWC, informed Dr. Hotze that he had just read a new book titled *Rapamycin, mTOR, Autophagy & Treating mTOR Syndrome* and said, "You have to read this book!"

After reading my book, Dr. Hotze ordered 600 copies of *Rapamycin, mTOR, Autophagy & Treating mTOR Syndrome*.

Dr. Hotze began his career as a conventional doctor, practicing emergency and family medicine. Over time, he began to realize that the drugs he was prescribing weren't helping his patients achieve robust health.

As a result, Dr. Hotze shifted his focus to allergy medicine, and in 1989, he opened the **Hotze Health &**

Wellness Center (HWC) as an allergy practice. Concurrent with this career change, Dr. Hotze began studying nutritional biochemistry to learn how vitamins, minerals, and other essential nutrients function in the body. He realized that a sound nutritional foundation is required for a healthy immune system and overall health.

Over the past 33 years, Hotze Health & Wellness Center, with its staff of over 70, has helped over 33,000 patients (whom Dr. Hotze calls "guests") obtain and maintain health and wellness naturally in an environment of extraordinary hospitality and guest services.

After reading my book, Dr. Hotze placed a call to me and we had a delightful conversation. He told me that he and several members of his staff had already started taking rapamycin, and they were beginning to recommend rapamycin to the guests at HWC. Dr. Hotze also invited me to be a guest on his Brighteon.TV program to share the story of rapamycin with his viewers.

HWC also has a compounding pharmacy Physicians Preference Pharmacy International or PPPI. Seeing an opportunity to educate other doctors about the anti-aging benefits of rapamycin, Dr. Hotze ordered those 600 copies of *Rapamycin, mTOR, Autophagy & Treating mTOR Syndrome*, and sent a copy to each of the 600 physicians who utilize the HWC compounding pharmacy. He also let them know PPPI could fill compounded rapamycin prescriptions for their patients.

Dr. Hotze and I share a passion for wanting to help people improve their health and the quality of their lives. I'm grateful that Dr. Hotze quickly understood the importance of rapamycin and that he purchased 600 copies of this book to distribute to physicians who will, in turn, begin to educate their patients about the health benefits of rapamycin.

Thank you, Dr. Hotze, for helping me to achieve my goal.

Let's Make Good Health Go Viral!

Appendix A

Rapamycin News Online Forum

Rapamycin News is simply the best online site for information related to rapamycin and its use as a longevity drug. The website is focused on providing practical, usable information to help people live longer and healthier lives. It is an online anti-aging-drug users' group with a news section and an active discussion forum. The site's primary focus is on all things related to rapamycin, but it also covers other drugs that are showing promise in animal and clinical studies, with reported benefits such as metformin, acarbose, SGLT2 inhibitors, and 17alpha-estradiol.

The site's news section covers important events in longevity-drug development, such as new animal and human clinical trials of drugs like rapamycin, as well as updates on these trials as they progress or are completed. The site is in frequent contact with leading rapamycin (and other longevity drug) researchers and is a conduit for new information on these drugs to the broader population of early adopters, longevity enthusiasts, and biohackers.

The discussion forum contains past and current discussions regarding everything related to rapamycin use, including how to get the best prices on rapamycin, a list of doctors that prescribe rapamycin, its interactions with other drugs and supplements to watch for, side effects and how to deal with them, and the benefits that people using rapamycin are experiencing.

The site has thousands of active users, including longtime rapamycin users, people just starting rapamycin, people who have not started taking rapamycin but want to learn more, physicians who utilize and prescribe rapamycin, and many of the top rapamycin scientists in the world.

The site is also actively working to move the state of longevity science forward by working closely with geroscientists (scientists studying the biology of aging). In early 2022, the site partnered with the University of Washington to help recruit for a survey-based longevity study of rapamycin users to get a better understanding of the results they are experiencing. Academic papers based on the data gathered from this study are expected to be published in 2023 and 2024. Other activities are ongoing and are announced on the website as they happen.

You can find Rapamycin Longevity News at the website www.rapamycin.news

About Rapamycin Longevity News

Based in the San Francisco Bay Area, Rapamycin Longevity News is a small group of technology professionals dedicated to healthier and longer lives through a good diet, regular exercise, and longevity medicines. They are advocates of geroscience research and greatly increased funding for the National Institute of Aging's Interventions Testing Program (ITP) and clinical trials of generic compounds showing promise.

Rapamycin is an FDA-approved drug that has been shown to increase lifespan and healthspan (typically by 15% to 30%) in every organism tested, from yeast to worms to mice. Doctors have, in the past few years, started to prescribe it to people off-label, and early adopters are testing it for themselves. In these forums we share our personal experiences and results with rapamycin and other anti-aging drugs. We are not doctors and no medical advice is given. This site is for informational purposes only

The main problems Rapamycin News is trying to address include the following:

Lack of a high-quality focused site for people interested in rapamycin. Right now, people who are trying rapamycin are scattered in small numbers on all kinds of websites without a critical mass of rapamycin users sharing their stories and perspectives over the long term. Here, we are trying to create a home for people interested in using the most promising anti-aging drugs and following the best, most current science related to age mitigation and healthy lifespan extension.

Geroscience researchers can't easily get access to the real-world evidence of rapamycin already being used in healthy populations. Right now, many researchers are very curious about rapamycin's use for anti-aging in healthy humans because it is so well proven in animals. But funding for clinical trials on generic longevity drugs is hard to come by. And, without the real-world evidence and human data from people's personal rapamycin trials, it's hard to move forward. Rapamycin News will share data with researchers, which will help everyone get better answers regarding the use of rapamycin and other prospective anti-aging medications. As the number of off-label rapamycin users grows, the data get better and better.

No clear FDA-approval path for rapamycin and similar anti-aging drugs. Currently, there is no clear path to FDA approval for drugs that can mitigate, slow, or reverse aging—especially for drugs like rapamycin, which are generic and inexpensive. Because the FDA doesn't recognize aging as a disease, and because the drug is off-patent, there is little or no money to be gained by a company funding a long and detailed clinical study of a drug like rapamycin for aging. The goal is to figure out a way to pull together the real-world evidence from off-label users of rapamycin and similar drugs. We will then try to build a large enough database of information on risks, benefits, and side effects in an effort to compel the FDA to seriously focus on this issue—or to get the NIH or other NGOs to fund these types of studies.

Raise awareness of anti-aging drugs and advocate for geroscience. It is unacceptable that the NIH puts so little investment (only about $300 million per year) into the basic biology of aging research, called The Division of Aging Biology, and its Interventions Testing Program. Most of the National Institute on Aging's budget goes into Alzheimer's disease research, not the fundamental causes of aging. The US government spends $6.5 billion per year for the National Cancer Institute, despite the fact that the biggest risk for cancer (and in fact almost all diseases) is aging. New research shows that the return on investment for public health is likely to exceed $38 trillion if rapamycin is effective in improving healthy lifespans by even a few years, which seems probable. There has to be much more public investment in the biology of aging research and Rapamycin News will continue to advocate for this.

I encourage everyone interested in rapamycin to regularly visit the Rapamycin News online forum.

Appendix B

AgelessRx & The PEARL Trial

AgelessRx is an online telemedicine longevity platform. It received **$485,000** in funding to initiate the PEARL trial in affiliation with the University of California. Funding for PEARL was obtained largely from a public crowdfunding campaign and presentations made by Bill Faloon, an Age Reversal Network co-founder, at scientific conferences urging attendees to donate. This is unique for two reasons. PEARL is apparently the first-ever crowdfunded human clinical trial. Also, the fact that the funding came from public donations is a testament to the widespread public interest in rapamycin as a drug that can improve healthspan and lifespan.

PEARL stands for the *Participatory Evaluation of Aging with Rapamycin for Longevity*. It is a double-blind, randomized, placebo-controlled trial designed to evaluate the safety and effectiveness of rapamycin for longevity in healthy adults.

The PEARL trial is important because it is the first nationwide telemedicine trial and the first large-scale intervention trial on longevity.

Study design: 150 healthy adults will be enrolled in this year-long trial. Two different doses of rapamycin will be tested. Participants will receive either 5 mg or 10 mg of rapamycin, or a placebo once weekly. Participants will receive multiple tests throughout the trial, valued at over $3,000. The tests include the latest **biological age testing** (methylation clocks), microbiome tests, **Dexa** body composition testing, **GlycanAge** testing, and blood panels with over 40 key blood markers. Ongoing medical evaluations will be provided to each participant.

Primary outcome measure: Changes in visceral fat as measured by Dexa scans.

Secondary outcomes: Range of clinical measures such as bone density and various blood test markers.

Principal investigators: James Watson, MD, and Sajad Zalzala, MD

The AgelessRx website is www.AgelessRx.com

Appendix C

Are We Getting the Biggest Bang for Our Buck?

Richard Miller is one of the site directors for the National Institutes on Aging's Intervention Testing Program (ITP). The image below, which is on his lab's website, emphasizes the importance of research into the biology of aging, and the potential for age- and disease-prevention drugs like rapamycin. This approach is dramatically different than the traditional "sick care" focus of the NIH and US medical system, in which they wait for disease to happen before initiating therapy.

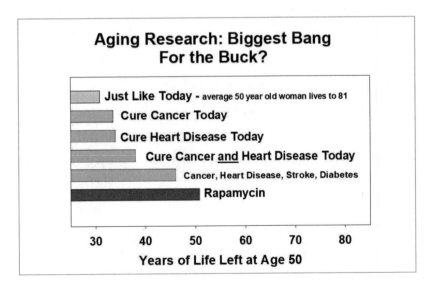

If rapamycin proves to be as effective in humans as it has been in mice, it will have a bigger impact than curing cancer, heart disease, stroke, and diabetes. This is because, even if these cures were found, there are many other diseases that people would succumb to. By comparison, the benefit of preventive, age-slowing strategies, which seem possible with rapamycin, would delay the onset all age-related diseases and potentially increase both healthspan and lifespan.

It is becoming increasingly obvious that the primary focus should be on the prevention of disease by slowing aging, rather than trying to treat a myriad of chronic degenerative diseases individually. The data clearly show that a healthcare system focused on prevention will provide the greatest benefit to the most people. The old adage "an ounce of prevention is worth a pound of cure" has been forgotten. Unfortunately, virtually all the NIH budget of $49 billion a year is spent on trying to "cure" individual diseases, while ignoring the fundamental role of prevention.

Most rapamycin users pay approximately $30 to $60 per month for their rapamycin, which is the copay on their insurance program. Over 20 years, this amounts to about $7,000 to $14,000. If the results seen in mice and other organisms transfers to humans, then we may achieve an additional 20 years of disease-free healthspan and lifespan. Compare that to the average cost of a single overnight stay in a hospital, which is about $13,600. The economic and social benefits are enormous.

If rapamycin keeps a person out of the hospital for just one day, then the healthcare system as a whole is at a break-even point. Annual healthcare expenditures in the United States are about $4.3 trillion. The potential for healthcare system savings with drugs like rapamycin are enormous. The savings are even more immediately realizable in developed countries that have national healthcare systems, including Canada, Japan, and the EU—every country except for the United States— because the single payer (the government) reaps the rewards (i.e., savings) from disease prevention.

The National Institute on Aging (NIA) sponsors the multi-institutional **Interventions Testing Program (ITP)**, to evaluate drugs and nutraceuticals that might slow aging and extend healthy lifespan in mice. The initial protocol focused on lifespan as the key endpoint. Agents that pass this screen are then evaluated in follow-up studies that include a wide range of age-sensitive tests, midlife pathology, and ideas about mechanism of effect. More information about the program can be found on the National Institute on Aging's ITP website. The site lists compounds tested or in progress, links to tissues that can be provided for collaborations, and information about how to submit a proposal to the ITP.

FREE Educational Resources from
The Natural Pharmacist

Never Stop Learning

Resource #1: In addition to rapamycin (plus exercise and a healthy diet), maintaining a healthy gut micro-biome is one of the most critical factors related to health and longevity. Bacterial imbalance in the gut microbiome causes many health problems and accel-erates biological aging. To emphasize this topic, I recently wrote a paper titled **"The Microbiome Theory of Aging"** which was published in the peer-reviewed medical journal *Integrative Medicine*. To get a copy of my article, do a search for the terms: **"imjournal Pelton Microbiome Theory of Aging"**

Resource #2: An article I wrote titled **"Postbiotic Metabolites: The New Frontier in Microbiome Science"** was published in the June 2019 issue of the *Townsend Letter*. This article will give you a good understanding of the importance of dietary fiber of and postbiotic metabolites. To read this article, do an Internet search for the following terms: **"Pelton Postbiotic Townsend"**

Resource #3: My article titled *Lactobacillus fermentum* ME-3: **A New Era in Glutathione Therapy**; published in June 2017 issue of *Townsend Letter*.

This article explains the wide-ranging health benefits of glutathione, including life extension. Plasma glutathione levels are now recognized as a reliable biomarker of aging. To read this article, do an Internet search for the following terms: **"Pelton Glutathione Townsend"**

Resource #4: Use the following link to Ross's website to get a FREE COPY of Ross's book titled: *Dr. Ohhira's Probiotics & Postbiotic Metabolites*: *The New Frontier in Microbiome Science*: https://naturalpharmacist. net/ohhirabook/

Resource #5: My article on **"Drug-Induced Nutrient Depletions"** (cover story in Nov. 2019 issue of the *Townsend Letter*). To get this article do an Internet search for: **"Pelton Townsend Depletions"**

Resource #6: Use the following link to get a FREE copy of my **"Quick Reference Guide to Drug-Induced Nutrient Depletions"**: https://www.naturalpharmacist.net/dind/

Resource #7: My article titled **"The Perfect Storm: Explaining the Loss of Microbiome Diversity and the Epidemic of Chronic Degenerative Diseases"**. Go to my blog at: www.naturalpharmacist.net/blog, scroll down and click on "Perfect Storm"

Resource #8: After writing *The Drug-Induced Nutrient Depletion Handbook*, I learned that oral contraceptives deplete more nutrients than any other class of drugs. This motivated me to write *The Pill Problem*, which teaches women how to avoid or correct the side effects from oral contraceptives. My book is available on Amazon.com. To read my article on this topic, published in the Sept. 2021 issue of the *Townsend Letter*, search for **"Pelton Townsend Pill"**.

Resource #9: Watch my 8-minute YouTube video titled **"Ross' Salad Buzz"**, which teaches people how to save time making salads with a diverse range of fiber-rich foods to feed your microbiome. Search for **"Ross Salad Buzz"**.

Resource #10: My 4.5-hour course titled *Natural Therapies for Depression and Anxiety* is hosted on the Udemy learning platform. To access this course, search for **"Pelton Udemy Depression"**.

Resource #11: Use the following link to get a FREE copy of my eBook titled *Let's Raise Healthy Kids*. Naturalpharmacist.net/kids

ABOUT THE AUTHOR

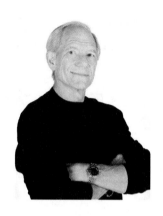

Ross Pelton, RPh, PhD, CCN is *The Natural Pharmacist*. His website, blog, and bio are at: www.naturalpharmacist.net.

Ross graduated from the University of Wisconsin in 1966 with a BS degree in pharmacy. In 1984 he earned his PhD in psychology from the University for Humanistic Studies in San Diego, CA. In 1994 he became a certified clinical nutritionist (CCN).

Ross was in the Peace Corps in Malaysia from 1971 to 1974 where he taught high school chemistry. From 1986 to 1994, Ross was hospital administrator of Hospital Santa Monica in Baja, Mexico, which was a facility that specialized in providing alternative, non-toxic cancer therapies. In 2011–2012, Ross was host of the radio talk show **Ask Dr. Ross** which aired on KCMX 880 AM News Talk Radio, in Medford, OR. From 2013 to 2016, Ross was a college professor at Southern Oregon University in Ashland, OR, where he and his wife Taffy taught a course on Psychopharmacology to master's degree students in the Counseling Psychology program. Ross has also been a member of Life Extension's Medical Advisory Board for over 20 years.

In October 1999, Ross was named one of the **Top 50 Most Influential Pharmacists in America** by

American Druggist magazine for his educational work in natural medicine.

Ross is the author of the following twelve books:

1. *Mind, Food, & Smart Pills* (Doubleday, 1988). Also translated into Italian.
2. *Alternatives in Cancer Therapy* (Simon & Schuster, 1994). Also translated into Italian and Chinese.
3. *How To Prevent Breast Cancer* (Simon & Schuster, 1995)
4. *The Drug-Induced Nutrient Depletion Handbook* (Lexi-Comp, 1999). 2nd edition published in 2001.
5. *The Nutritional Cost of Prescription Drugs* (Morton Publishing, 2000)
6. *The Natural Therapeutics Pocket Guide* (Lexi-Comp, 2000)
7. *The Nutritional Cost of Drugs, 2nd Edition* (Lexi-Comp, 2001)
8. *Natural Therapies to Prevent and Treat Viral Infections* (eBook 2010)
9. *Let's Have Healthy Kids* (eBook 2010)
10. *The Pill Problem* (paperback & eBook 2013)
11. *Dr. Ohhira's Probiotics & Postbiotic Metabolites: The New Frontier in Microbiome Science* (2020)
12. *Rapamycin, mTOR & Autophagy & Treating mTOR Syndrome* (2021)

Ross lives with his wife Taffy in Ashland, OR. Since 2014, Ross has been the Scientific Director for Dallas-based Essential Formulas Incorporated (EFI) **www.essentialformulas.com**. As the Scientific Director at EFI, Ross has played a major role in educating the world about the importance of postbiotic metabolites, which are compounds that probiotic bacteria produce when they ferment dietary fiber in the colon. Postbiotic metabolites are now being recognized as master health-regulating compounds that influence every organ system in the body.

ACKNOWLEDGMENTS

Thanks to Bill Faloon and Life Extension www.lef.org

Thank you, Bill Faloon, co-founder of the Life Extension Foundation, for introducing me to rapamycin. I joined the Life Extension group in 1980 when the organization was founded by you and Saul Kent. Now, over four decades later, Life Extension's research team and their monthly Life Extension magazine remain one of my most valuable sources of cutting-edge information on the science and technology of life extension. I have also been a member of Life Extension's Medical Advisory Board for over 20 years.

My rapamycin journey began when I attended Bill Faloon's presentation at the 2017 RAADfest conference in Las Vegas. **RAAD** stands for **Revolution Against Aging & Death**. Faloon summarized studies conducted in animals reporting that rapamycin produces improvements in health, delayed onset of diseases, and could promote significant life extension.

My obsession with rapamycin accelerated in early 2021 after I listened to several episodes of Peter Attia,

MD's *The Drive* podcast. Peter interviewed scientists who played key roles in the rapamycin/mTOR story including David Sabatini, Joan Mannick, Matt Kaeberlein and Lloyd Klickstein. My background in pharmacy and science and my decades-long passion regarding all things related to health suddenly ignited a "rapamycin fire" in me. Most of the information about rapamycin, mTOR & autophagy is in scientific journals. I realized that this story needed to be communicated to the general public and that's how I got started on this journey.

I encourage people who are interested in health and specifically, healthy longevity, to join the Life Extension group. In addition to gaining access to affordable high quality, cutting-edge nutritional supplements, you will also receive the monthly *Life Extension* magazine, which will keep you updated on advances related to disease risk reduction and the deceleration of biological aging.

To obtain a complimentary subscription to *Life Extension Magazine*, go to: www.LifeExtension.com/free or call 1-800-226-2370 (24 hours).

REFERENCES

1   Harrison DE, et al. Rapamycin fed late in life extends lifespan in genetically heterogeneous mice. *Nature*. 2009 Jul 16;460(7253):392-5.

2   McCay CM, et al. The effect of retarded growth upon the length of life span and upon the ultimate body size. 1935. *Nutrition*. 1989, 5: 155-71.

3   Lashinger LM, et al. Rapamycin partially mimics the anticancer effects of calorie restriction in a murine model of pancreatic cancer. *Cancer Prev Res*. July 2011;4:1041-101.

4   Ye Lan, et al. Rapamycin has a biphasic effect on insulin sensitivity in C2C12 myotubes due to sequential disruption of mTORC1 and mTORC2. *Front Genet* 2012 Sep 11;3:177.

5   Mondesire WH, et al. Targeting Mammalian Target of Rapamycin Synergistically Enhances Chemotherapy-Induced Cytotoxicity in Breast Cancer Cells. *Clinical Cancer Research*. 2004 Oct 15;10(20:7031-42.

6   Bjedov I, et al. Mechanisms of Life Span Extension by Rapamycin in the Fruit Fly Drosophila melanogaster. *Cell Metab*. 2010 Jan 6;11(1):35-46.

7   ClinicalTrials.gov. Participatory Evaluation (of) Aging (with) Rapamycin (for) Longevity Study. https://clinicaltrials.gov/ct2/show/NCT04488601

8   Miller RA, et al. Rapamycin, but not resveratrol or simvastatin, extends life span of genetically heterogeneous mice. *The journals of gerontology Series A, Biological sciences and medical sciences*. 2011;66(2):191–201.

9   Miller RA, et al. Rapamycin-mediated lifespan increase in mice is dose and sex dependent and metabolically distinct from dietary restriction. *Aging Cell*. 2014;13(3):468–477.

10 Blagosklonny MV. Aging and immortality: quasi-programmed senescence and its pharmacologic inhibition. *Aging (Albany NY)*. 2019 Oct 15(11(19):8048-8067.

11 Blagosklonny MV An anti-aging drug today: from senescence-promoting genes to anti-aging pill. *Drug Discov Today*. 2007 Mar; 12(5-6):218-24.

12 Mannick JB. mTOR inhibition improves immune function in the elderly. *Sci Transl Med*. 2014 Dec 24;6(268):268ra179.

13 Chang GR, et al. Long-term Administration of Rapamycin Reduces Adiposity, but Impairs Glucose Tolerance in High-Fat Diet-fed KK/HIJ Mice. Basic Clin *Pharmacol Toxicol*. 2009 Sept;105(3):188-98.

14 Halford B. Rapamycin's secrets unearthed. *Chemical & engineering News*. July 18, 2016'94(29).

15 Gerber K. Rapamycin's Resurrection: A New Way to Target the Cancer Cell Cycle. *J Natl Ca Inst*. 17 Oct 2001;93(20):1517-1519.

16 Lu JY, et al. Comparative transcriptomics reveals circadian and pluripotency networks as two pillars of longevity regulation. *Cell Metab*. 022 Jun 7;34z96):836-856.e5.

17 Gorbunova V. From long-lived animal species to human interventions. Healthy Longevity webinar and personal communication with Dr. Gorbunova.

18 Sudarsanam S and Johnson DE. Functional consequences of mTOR inhibition. *Curr Opin Drug Discov Devel*. 2010 Jan;13(1):31-40.

19 Masoro EJ. Dietary restriction-induced life extension: a broadly based biological phenomenon. *Biogerontology*. 2006;7(3):153-155

20 Everitt AV and Le Couteur DG. Life extension by calorie restriction in humans. *Ann N Y Acad Sci*. 2007 Oct;1114:428-33.

21 Brown EJ, et al. A mammalian protein targeted by G1-arresting rapamycin-receptor complex". *Nature*. June 1994;369 (6483): 756–8.

22 Sabatini DM, et al. RAFT1: a mammalian protein that binds to FKBP12 in a rapamycin-dependent fashion and is homologous to yeast TORs. *Cell*. July 1994;78 (1): 35–43.

23 Sabers CJ, et al. Isolation of a protein target of the FKBP12-rapamycin complex in mammalian cells. *J Biol Chem*. Jan 1995;270(2):815-22.

24 Press Release: 2016 Nobel Prize in Physiology or Medicine.

25 Stroikin Y, et al. Testing the "garbage" accumulation theory of ageing: mitotic activity protects cells from death induced by inhibition of autophagy. *Biogerontology*. 2005 Jan;6:39-47.

26 Glick D, at al. Autophagy: cellular and molecular mechanisms. *J Pathol*. 2010;221(1):3-12.

27 Fang Y, et al. Signaling pathways and mechanisms of hypoxia-induced autophagy in the animal cells. *Cell Biol Int*. 2015 Aug;39(8):891-8.

28 Scherz-Shouval R, et al. Reactive oxygen species are essential for autophagy and specifically regulate the activity of Atg4. *EMBO J*. 2007 Apr 4;26(7):1749-60.

29 Deleyto-Seladas N and Efeyan A. The mTOR-Autophagy Axis and the Control of Metabolism. *Front Cell Dev Biol*. 2021 Jul 1;9:655731.

30 Kim YC and Guan KL. mTOR: a pharmacologic target for autophagy regulation. *J Clin Invest*. Jan 2, 2015;125(1):25-32.

31 Bareja A, et al. Maximizing Longevity and Healthspan: Multiple Approaches All Converging on Autophagy. *Front Cell Dev Biol*. 2019 Sep 6;7(183).

32 Cota D, et. al. Hypothalamic mTOR Signaling Regulates Food Intake. *Science*. 2006 May 12;312(5775):927-930.

33 Vijayakumar K. Autophagy: An evolutionarily conserved process in the maintenance of stem cells and aging. *Cell Biochemistry and Function*. 2019;37(6).

34 Hall MN. mTOR-what does it do? *Transplantation Proceedings*. 2008 Dec;40(10 Suppl):S5-S8.

35 Kourtis N and Tavernarakis N. Autophagy and cell death in model organisms. *Cell Death & Differentiation*. 2009 Jan;16(1):21-30.

36 Swindell WR. Dietary restriction in rats and mice: A meta-analysis and review of the evidence for genotype-dependent effects on lifespan. *Ageing Res Rev*. 2012 Apr;11(2):254-270.

37 Masoro EJ. Dietary restriction-induced life extension: a broadly based biological phenomenon. *Biogerontology*. 2006;7(3):153-155.

38 Bodkin NL, et al. Mortality and morbidity in laboratory-maintained Rhesus monkeys and effects of long-term dietary restriction. *J Gerontol A Biol Sci Med Sci*. 2003;58(3):212-219.

39 Anton SD, et al. Caloric Restriction to Moderate Senescence: Mechanisms and Clinical Utility. *Curr Transl Geriatr Exp Gerontol Rep*. 2013 Dec 13;2(4):239-246.

40 Johnson JB, et al. Alternate day calorie restriction improves clinical findings and reduces markers of oxidative stress and inflammation in overweight adults with moderate asthma. *Free Radic Biol Med*. 2007;42:665–674.

41 Eaton SB, et al. Stone agers in the fast lane: chronic degenerative diseases in evolutionary prespective. *Am J Med*. 1988 Apr;84(4):739-49.

42 Falcon LJ and Harris-Love,MO. Sarcopenia and the New ICD-10=CM Code: Screening, Staging, and Diagnosis Considerations. *Fed Pract*.2017 Jul;34(7):24-32.

43 Koller M. Sarcopenia-a geriatric pandemic: A narrative review. *Wien Med Wochenschr*. 2022 Apr 13. https://pubmed.ncbi.nlm.nih.gov/35416610/

44 Rosenberg I. Summary comments: epidemiological and methodological problems in determining nutritional status of older persons. *Am J Clin Nutr*. 1989;50:1231–3.

45 Evans W, et al. Biomarkers: The 10 Keys to Prolonging Vitality. New York, Fireside, 1991.

46 Fiatarone MA, et al. High-Intensity Strength Training in Nonagenarians: Effects on Skeletal Muscle. *JAMA*. 1990;263(22):3029-3034.

47 Sports and exercise among Americans. https://www.bls.gov/opub/ted/2016/sports-and-exercise-among-americans.htm

48 Bhopatkar AA, et al. Disorder and cysteines in proteins: A design for orchestration of conformational see-saw and modulatory functions. *Prog Mol Biol Transl Sci*. 2020;174:331-373.

49 Alberts B, et al. Molecular Biology of the Cell. 4th edition. New York: Garland· Science; 2002. *The Shape and Structure of Proteins*. Available from: https://www.ncbi.nlm.nih.gov/books/NBK26830/

50 Breen L and Phillips SM. Skeletal muscle protein metabolism in the elderly: Interventions to counteract the 'anabolic resistance' of aging. *Nutrition & Metabolism*. 2011 Oct 5;8:68.

51 Grimby G, Saltin B. The ageing muscle. *Clin Physiol*. 1983. 3:209–218.

52 Hughes VA, Frontera WR, Wood M, et al. Longitudinal muscle strength changes in older adults: influence of muscle mass, physical activity, and health. *J Gerontol A Biol Sci Med Sci*. 2001. 56:B209–B217.

53 Breen L and Phillips SM. Skeletal muscle protein metabolism in the elderly: Interventions to counteract the 'anabolic resistance; of aging. *Nutr Metab (Lond)*. 2011 Oct 5;8:68.

54 Chapman IM. Endocrinology of anorexia of ageing. *Best Pract Res Clin endocrinol Metab*. 2004;18(3):437-452.

55 Wysokinski A, et al. Mechanisms of the anorexia of aging—a review. *Age (Dordr)*. 2015 Aug;37(4):81.

56 Soenen S and Chapman IM. Body weight, anorexia, and undernutrition in older people. *J Am Med Dir Assoc*. 2013 Sep;14(9):642-8.

57 Paddon-Jones D, et al. Differential stimulation of muscle protein synthesis in elderly humans following isocaloric ingestion of amino acids or whey protein. *Exp Gerontol*. 2006;41:215–219.

58 Walrand S, et al. Functional impact of high protein intake on healthy elderly people. *Am J Physiol Endocrinol Metab*. 2008 Oct;295(4):E921-E928.

59 Volpi E, et al. Is the optimal level of protein intake for older adults greater than the recommended dietary allowance? *J Gerontol A Biol Sci Med Sci*. 2013;68:677-81.

60 Bauer J, et al. Evidence-based recommendations for optimal dietary protein intake in older people: a position paper from the PROT-AGE Study Group. *J Am Med Dir Assoc*. 2013 Aug 1;14(8):542-59.

61 Nowson C and O'Connell S. Protein Requirements and Recommendations for Older People: A Review. *Nutrients*. 2015 Aug;7(8):6874-6899.

62 Phillips SM, et al. Protein "requirements" beyond the RDA: implications for optimizing health. *Applied Physiology, Nutrition, and Metabolism*. 2016;41(5):565-72.

63 Berrazaga I, Micard V, Gueugneau M, et al. The Role of the Anabolic Properties of Plant- versus Animal-Based Protein Sources in Supporting Muscle Mass Maintenance: A Critical Review. *Nutrients*. 2019;11(8):1825.

64 Drummond MJ and Rasmussen BB. Leucine-Enriched Nutrients and the Regulation of mTOR Signaling and Human Skeletal Muscle Protein Synthesis. *Curr Opin clin Nutr Metab Care*. 2008 May;11(3):222-226.

65 Van Vliet S, et al. the Skeletal Muscle Anabolic Response to Plant- versus Animal-Based protein Consumption. *Journal of Nutrition*. 2015 Jul;145(9):1981-91.

66 Jager R, et al. International Society of Sports Nutrition Position Stand: protein and exercise. *J Int Soc Sports Nutr*. 2017 Jun 20;14:20.

67 Lee SY, et al. Effects of leucine-rich protein supplements in older dults with sarcopenia: A systematic review and meta-analysis of randomized controlled trials. *Arch Gerontol Geriatr*. 2022 Sep-Oct;102:104758.

68 Giallauria F, et al. Resistance training and sarcopenia. *Monaldi Arch Chest Dis*. 2016;84(1-2):738. doi: 10.4081/monaldi.2015.738.

69 Chen N, et al. Effects of resistance training in healthy older people with sarcopenia: a systematic review and meta-analysis of randomized controlled trials. *Eur Rev Aging Phys Act*. 2021'18:23.

70 Tipton KD, et al. Assessing the Role of Muscle Protein Breakdown in Response to Nutrition and Exercise in Humans. *Sports Med*. 2018;48(Suppl 1):53-64.

71 Norton L, et al. The Leucine content of complete meal directs peak activation but not duration of skeletal muscle protein synthesis and mammalian target of rapamycin signaling in rats. *J Nutr*. 2009, 139 (6): 1103-1109.

72 Devries MC and Phillips SM. Supplemental Protein in Support of Muscle Mass and Health: Advantage Whey. *J Food Sci*. 2015 Mar;80 Suppl 1:A8-A15.

73 Nobukuni T, et al. Amino acids mediate mTOR/raptor signaling through activation of class 3 phosphatidylinositol 3OH-kinase. *Proc Natl Acad Sci USA*. 2005, 102: 14238-14243.

74 Bjedov I, et al. Increased fidelity of protein synthesis extends lifespan. *Cell Metabolism*. 2021 Nov 2;33(11):2288-2300.

75 Lamming, D. Rapamycin and Rapalogs. *Preprints* 2021, 2021020491.

76 Kennedy BK and Lamming DW. The mechanistic Target of Rapamycin: The grand conductor of metabolism and aging. *Cell Metab*. 2016 Jun 14;23(6):990-1003.

77 Beauchamp EM and Platanias LC. The evolution of the TOR pathway and its role in cancer. *Oncogene*. 2013;32:3923-3932.

78 Dancey J. mTOR signaling and drug development in cancer. *Nat Rev Clin Oncol*. 2010 Apr;7(4):209-19.

79 Law BK. Rapamycin: an anti-cancer immunosuppressant? *Crit Rev Oncol Hematol*. 20015 Oct;56(1):47-60.

80 Sherston SN, et al. Predictors of Cancer Risk in the Long-Germ Solid-Organ Transplant Recipient. *Transplantation*. 2014 Mar 27;97(6):605-611.

81 United Network for Organ Sharing. 2021. https://unos.org/news/deceased-organ-donation-and-transplant-annual-trend-continues-2020/

82 Tessari G and Girolomoni G. Nonmelanoma Skin Cancer in Solid Organ Transplant Recipients: Update on Epidemiology, Risk Factors, and Management. *Dermatologic Surgery*. Oct 2012;38(10):1622-1630.

83 Alter M, et al. Non-melanoma skin cancer is reduced after switch of immunosuppression to mTOR-inhibitors in organ transplant recipients. *J Dtsch Dermatol Ges*. 2014 Jun;12(6):480-8.

84 iData Research. https://idataresearch.com/stents-implanted-per-year-in-the-u-s/

85 Chisari A, et al. The Ultimaster Biodegradable-Polymer Sirolimus_Eluting Stent: An Updated Review of Clinical Evidence. *Int J Mil Sci*. 2016;17(9):1490.

86 Lesniewski LA, et al. Dietary rapamycin supplementation reverses age-related vascular dysfunction and oxidative stress, while modulating nutrient-sensing, cell cycle, and senescence pathways. *Aging Cell.* 2017;16(1):17-26.

87 Lips DJ, et al. Molecular determinants of myocardial hypertrophy and failure: alternative pathways for beneficial and maladaptive hypertrophy. *Eur. Heart J.* 2003;24:883-896.

88 Gu J, et al. Rapamycin Inhibits Cardiac Hypertrophy by Promoting Autophagy via MEK/ERK/Beclin-1 Pathway. *Front Physiol.* 2016 Mar 18;7:104.

89 Gao G, et al. Rapamycin regulated the balance between cardiomyocyte apoptosis and autophagy in chronic heart failure by inhibition mTOR signaling. *Int J Mil Med.* 2020 Jan;45(1):195-209.

90 Zhu F. Neuroprotective effect of rapamycin against Parkinson's disease in mice. *Journal of Zhejiang University.* 2018 May 25;47(5):465-472.

91 Spillman P. et al. Inhibition of mTOR by rapamycin abolishes cognitive deficits and reduces amyloid-beta levels in a mouse model of Alzheimer's disease. *PLoS* One. 2010 Apr 1;5(4):e9979.

92 Bagherpour B, et al. Promising effect of rapamycin on multiple sclerosis. Mult Scler Relat Disord. 2018 Nov;26:40-45.

93 Wen HY, et al. Low-Dose Sirolimus Immunoregulation Therapy in Patients with Active Rheumatoid Arthritis: A 24-Week Follow-up of the Randomized, Open-Label, Parallel-controlled Trial. *J Immunol Res.* 2019 Nov 3;2019:7684352.

94 Piranavan P and Peri A. Improvement of renal and non-renal SLE outcome measures on sirolimus therapy - A 21-year follow-up study of 73 patients. *Clin Immunol.* 2021 Aug;229:108781.

95 Callahan EA editor. Current Status and Response to the Global Obesity Pandemic: Proceedings of a workshop. 2019 Jun 25. https://pubmed.ncbi.nlm.nih.gov/31334935/

96 Fryar CD, et al., Prevalence of Overweight, Obesity, and Severe Obesity Among Adults Aged 20 and Over: United States, 1960-1962 Through 2017-2018. https://www.cdc.gov/nchs/data/hestat/obesity-adult-17-18/obesity-adult.htm

97 Hwangbo DS, et al. Mechanisms of Lifespan Regulation by Calorie Restriction and Intermittent Fasting in Model Organisms. *Nutrients* 2020;12(4):1194.

98 Roth LS and Polotsky AJ. Can we live longer by eating less: A review of caloric restriction and longevity. *Maturitas.* 2012 Apr;71(4):315-319.

99 Most J, et al. Calorie restriction in humans: an update. *Ageing Res Rev.* 2017 Oct;39:36-45.

100 Stunkard, AJ, et al. The results of treatment for obeity. *Arch Intern Med.* 1959;103:79-85.

101 Deblon N, et al. Chronic mTOR inhibition by rapamycin induces muscle insulin resistance despite weight loss in rats. *Br J Pharmacol*. 2012 Aapr;165(7):2325-2340.

102 Rovira J, et al. Effect of mTOR inhibitor on body weight: from an experimental rat model to human transplant patients. *Transpl Int*. 2008 Oct;21(10):992-8.

103 Scarpace PJ, et al. Rapamycin Normalizes Serum Leptin by Alleviating Obesity and Reducing Leptin Synthesis in Aged Rats. *J Gerontol A Biol Sci Med Sci*. 2016 Jul;71(7):891-9.

104 Toutouzas K, et al. Sirolimus-eluting stents: a review of experimental and clinical findings. *Z Karkiol*. 2002;91 Suppl 3:49-57.

105 Boada C, et al. Rapamycin-Loaded Biomimetic Nanoparticles Reverse Vascular Inflammation. *Circulation Research*. 2020;126:25-37.

106 Nhuyen QD, et al. Noninfectious Uveitis: Evolution through Preclinical and Clinical Studies. *Ophthalmology*. 2018 Dec;125(12):1984-19+93.

107 Shen G, et al. Mammalian target of rapamycin as a therapeutic target in osteoporosis. *J Cell Physiol*. 2018 May;233(5):3929-3944.

108 Yin ZY, et al. Rapamycin facilitates fracture healing through inducing cell autophagy and suppressing cell apoptosis in bone tissues. *Eur Med Pharmacol Sci*. 2017 Nov;21(21):4989-4998.

109 Yang GE, et al. Rapamycin-induced autophagy activity promotes fracture healing in rats. *Eur Ther Med*. 2015 Oct;10(4):1327-1333.

110 Martin SA, et al. Rapamycin impairs bone accrual nin young adult mice independent of Nrf2. *Exp Gerontol*. 2021 Aug 10;111516.

111 Hussein O, et al. Rapamycin inhibits osteolysis and improves survival in a model of experimental bone metastases. *Cancer Letters*. 2012 Jan;414(2):176-84.

112 Gambacurta A, et al. Human osteogenic differentiation in Space: proteomic and epigenetic clues to better understand osteoporosis. *Sci Rep*. 2019 Jun 6;9(1):8343.

113 Bari M, Battista N, Merlini G, et al. The SERiSM project: preliminary data on human stem cell reprogramming in microgravity. *Frontiers in Physiology*. 2018;9.

114 Luo D, et al. Rapamycin reduces severity of senile osteoporosis by activating osteocyte Autophagy. *Osteoporosis International*. 2016;27:1093-1101.

115 Wang L, et al. Male rodent model of age-related bone loss in men. *Bone*. 2001;29(2):141-148.

116 Kuo D, et al. Rapamycin reduces severity of senile osteoporosis by activating osteocyte autophagy. *Osteoporosis International*. 2016;27:1093-1101.

117 Li XN, et al. Rapamycin activates autophagy by inhibition mTOR pathway to alleviate early osteoporosis in rats with skeletal fluorosis. *Chinese Journal of Industrial Hygiene and Occupational Diseases*. 2021 May 20;39(5):321-327.

118 Altschuler RA, et al. Tapamycin Added to Diet in Late Mid-Life Delays Age-Related Hearing Loss in UMHET4 Mice. *Front Cell Neurosci.* 2021 Apr 7;15:658972.

119 Hosoya M, et al. Estimating the concentration of therapeutic range using disease-specific iPS cells: Low-dose rapamycin therapy for Pendred syndrome. *Regen Ther.* 2018 Dec 17;10:54-63.

120 Dhadse P, et al. The link between periodontal disease and cardiovascular disease: How far we have come in the last two decades? *J Indian Soc Periodotol.* 2010 Jul-Sep;14(3):148-154.

121 Scannapieco F, et al. Associations between periodontal disease and risk for nosocomial bacterial pneumonia and chronic obstructive pulmonary disease. A systematic review. *Ann Periodontal.* 2003 Dec;8(1):54-69.

122 Beydoun MA, et al. Clinical and Bacterial Markers of Periodontitis and Their Association with Incident All-Cause and Alzheimer's Disease Dementia in a Large National Survey. *J Alzheimer's Dis.* 2020;75(1):157-172.

123 Nazir MA. Prevalance of periodontal disease, its association with systemic diseases and prevention. *Int J Health Sci (Qassim).* 2017 Apr-Jun;11(2):72-80.

124 Ebersole JL, et al. Aging, inflammation, immunity and periodontal disease. *Periodontol.* 2000 Oct;72(1):54-75.

125 An JY, et al. Rapamycin rejuvenates oral health in aging mice. *Elife.* 2020 Apr 28;9:e54318

126 Kolosova NG, et al. Prevention of age-related macular degeneration-like retinopathy by rapamycin in rats. *Am J Pathol.* 2012 Aug;181(2):472-7.

127 Niu Z, et al. Protective effect of rapamycin in models of retinal degeneration. *Exp Eye Res.* 2021 Sep;210:108700.

128 Su W, et al. Rapamycin is neuroprotective in a rat chronic hypertensive glaucoma model. *PLoS* One. 2014 Jun 12;9(6):e99719.

129 Harder JM, et al. Disturbed glucose and pyruvate metabolism in glaucoma with neuroprotection by pyruvate or rapamycin. *Proc Natl Acad Sci USA.* 2020 Dec 29;117(52):33619-33627.

130 DeKlotz CMC, et al. Dramatic improvement of facial angiofibromas in tuberous sclerosis with topical rapamycin: optimizing a treatment protocol. *Arch Dermatil.* 2011 Sep;147(9):1116-7.

131 Wheless JW, et al. A Novel Topical Rapamycin Cream for the Treatment of Facial Angiofibromas in Tuberous Sclerosis Complex. *J Child Neurology.* 2013 Jul;28(7):933-6.

132 Burger C, et al. Blocking mTOR Signalling with Rapamycin Ameliorates Imiquimod-induced Psoriasis in Mice. *Acta Derm Venereol.* 2017 Oct 2;97(9):1087-1094.

133 Ekici Y, et al. Effect of rapamycin on would healing: an experimental study. *Transplant Proc.* 2007 May;39(4):1201-3.

134 Costa-Mattioli M, Monteggia LM. mTOR complexes in neurodevelopmental and neuropsychiatric disorders. *Nat Neurosci* 2013; 16: 1537–1543.

135 Ricciardi S, et al. Reduced AKT/mTOR signaling and protein synthesis dysregulation in a Rett syndrome animal model. *Hum Mol Genet* 2011; 20: 1182–1196.

136 Oddo S. The role of mTOR signaling in Alzheimer disease. *Front Biosci* 2012; 4: 941–952.

137 Spilman, P., Podlutskaya, N., Hart, M. J., Debnath, J., Gorostiza, O., Bredesen, D., et al. (2010). Inhibition of mTOR by rapamycin abolishes cognitive deficits and reduces amyloid-β levels in a mouse model of Alzheimer's disease. *PLoS One* 5:e9979.

138 Blagosklonny MV. Rapamycin for longevity: opinion article. *Aging (Albany NY)*. 2019 Oct 15;11(19):8048-8067.

139 Bitto A, et al. Transient rapamycin treatment can increase lifespan and healthspan in middle-aged mice. *eLife*. 2016; Aug 23;5:e16351.

140 Johnson SC, et al. Dose-dependent effects of mTOR inhibition on weight and mitochondrial disease in mice. *Front Genet*. 2015; 6:247.

141 Taylor DH, et al. Benefits of smoking cessation for longevity. *Am J Public Health*. 2002; 92:990–96.

142 Selvin E, et al. Prevalence and risk factors for erectile dysfunction in the US. *Am J Med*. 2007 Feb;120(2):151-7.

143 Kouidrat Y, et al. High prevalence of erectile dysfunction in diabetes: a systematic review and meta-analysis of 145 studies. *Diabet Med*. 2017 Sep;34(9):1185-1192.

144 Kaya E, Sikka SC, Gur S. A comprehensive review of metabolic syndrome affecting erectile dysfunction. *J Sex Med*. 2015;12:856–875.

145 Kloner R. Erectile dysfunction and hypertension. *Int J Impot Res*. 2007 May-Jun;19(3):296-302.

146 Lin H, et al. Rapamycin Supplementation May Ameliorate Erectile Function in Rats With Streptozotocin-Induced Type 1 Diabetes by Inducing Autophagy and Inhibiting Apoptosis, Endothelial Dysfunction, and Corporal Fibrosis. *J. Sex Med*. 2018 S?ep;15(9):1246-1259.

147 Lagoda G, et al. FK506 and rapamycin neuroprotect erection and involve different immunophilins in a rat model of cavernous nerve injury. *J Sex Med*. 2009 Jul;6(7):1914-23.

148 La Favor, JD, et al. Rapamycin Suppresses Penile NADPH Oxidase Activity to Preserve Erectile Function in Mice Fed a Westen Style High-Fat, High-Sucrose Diet. *Biomedicines*. 2021 Dec 30;10(1):68.

149 KAY HH. Pregnancy before Age 20 Years and after Age 35 Years. Chapter 54 in *Clinical Obstetrics: The Fetus & Mother, Third Edition*. Editors Feece A and Hobbins JC. 2007 Jan 1. https://onlinelibrary.wiley.com/doi/abs/10.1002/9780470753293.ch54

150 Cheng Y, et al. Promotion of Ovarian Follicle Growth following mTOR Activation: Synergistic Effects of AKT Stimulators. *PLOS One.* 2015 Feb 24:1-9.

151 Guo J, et al. Oocyte stage-specific efforts of mTOR determine granulosa cell fate and oobyte quality in mice. *Proc Natl Acad Sci USA.* 2018;115:E5326-33.

152 Roa J, et al. The mammalian target of rapamycin as novel central regulatory of pubery onset via modulation of jypothalamic kiss1 system. *Endocrinology.* 2009;150:5016-26.

153 Zhang XM, et al. Rapamycin preserves the follicle pool reserve and prolongs the ovarian lifespan of female rats via modulatin mTOR activation and sirtuin expression. *Gene.* 2013;523:82-7.

154 Dou X, et al. Short-term rapamycin treatment increases ovarian lifespan in young and middle-aged female mice. *Aging Cell.* 2017 May 22;16(4):825-836.

155 Tang H, et al. Rapamycin protects aging muscle. *Aging (Albany NY).* 2019 Aug 31;11(16):5868-5870.

156 Blagosklonny MV. Aging and immortality: quasi-programmed senescence and its pharmacologic inhibition. *Cell Cycle.* 2006; 5:2087–102.

157 Wang H, et al. Mammalian target of rapamycin inhibitor RAD001 sensitizes endometrial cancer cells into paclitaxel-induced apoptosis via the induction of autophagy. *Oncol Lett.* 2016 Dec. 12(6):5029-5035.

158 Coppock JF, et al. mTOR inhibition as an adjuvant therapy in a metastatic model of HPV+ HNSCC. *Oncotarget.* 2016 Apr 26;7(17):24228-41.

159 Perk J. Non-communicable diseases, a growing threat to global health. *European Society of Cardiology.* 2017 Aug 30;15(14).

160 Shih YC and Hurria A. Preparing for an epidemic: cancer care in an aging population. *Am Soc Clin Oncol Edu Book.* 2014:133-7.

161 Ounpuu S, et al. The impending global epidemic of cardiovascular diseases. *Eur Heart J.* 2000 Jun;21(11):880-803.

162 Malmborg P and Hildebrand H. The emerging global epidemic of pediatric inflammatory bowel disease-causes and consequences. *J Intern Med.* 2016 Mar;279(3):241-58.

163 Saklayen MG. The Global Epidemic of the Metabolic Syndrome. *Curr Hypertens Rep.* 2018 Feb 26;20(2):12.

164 Kim R. et al. Understanding the obesity epidemic. *BMJ.* 2019 Jul 3;366:14409.

165 New M. Arthritis: an impending public health epidemic. *J Okla State Med Assoc.* 2001 Feb;94(2):63-64.

166 Lee TS and Krishnan KR. Alzheimer's disease-the inexorable epidemic. *Ann Acad Med Singapore.* 2019 Jul;39(7):505-2.

167 Graf WE. Et al. The autism "epidemic": Ethical, legal, and social issues in a developmental spectrum disorder. *Neurology.* 2017 Apr 4;88(14):1371-1380.

168 Lardizabal A. Is financial gain to blame for the growing ADHD epidemic? *J Child Adolesc Psychiatr Nurs.* 2012 Aug;25(3):164.

169 NAFLD-NASH:An Under-Recognized Epidemic. *Curr Vasc Pharmacol.* 2018;16(3):209-213.

170 Tucci V and Moukaddam N. We are the hollow men: The worldwide epidemic of mental illness, psychiatric and behavioral emergencies, and its impact on patients and providers. *J Emerg Trauma Shock.* 2017 Jan-Mar;10(1):4-6.

171 Blagosklonny MV. Rapamycin for longevity: opinion article. *Aging (Albany NY).* 2019 Oct 15;11(19):8048-8067.

172 Lins Vieira RF. Et al. Exercise activates AMPK signaling: Impact on glucose uptake in the skeletal muscle in aging. *J Rehab Therapy.* Aug 4, 2020;2(2):48-53.

173 Ashrafizadeh M. et al. Autophagy regulation using luteolin: new insight into its anti-tumor activity. *Cancer Cell Int.* 2020 Nov 4;20(1):537.

174 Theoharides TC, et al. Brain "fog" inflammation and obesity: key aspects of neuropsychiatric disorders improved by luteolin. *Front Neurosci.* 2 July 2015;9:225.

175 Makhov P, et al. Piperlongumine promotes autophagy via inhibition of Akt/mTOR signaling and mediates cancer cell death. *British Journal of Cancer.* Jan 16, 2014;110:899-907.

176 Aggarwal BB and Harikumar KB. *Int J Biochem & Cell Biology.* Jan 2009;41(1):40-59.

177 Guo S, et al. Curcumin activates autophagy and attenuates oxidative damage in EA.hy926 cells via the Akt/mTOR pathway. *Mol Med Rep.* 2016 Mar13(3):2187-93.

178 Shen L, et al. Curcumin and aging. Biofactors. Jan-Feb 2013;39(1):133-40.

179 Amamd P, et al. Bioavailability of Curcumin: Problems and Promises. *Mol. Pharmaceutics.* 14 Nov 2007;4, 6, 807–818.

180 Kumar D, et al. Enhanced bioavailability and relative distribution of free (unconjugated) curcuminoids following the oral administration of a food-grade formulation with fenugreek dietary fibre: A randomized double-blind crossover study. *J Functional Foods.* 2016 Apr;22:578-587.

181 Lee HS. *Gynostemma Pentaphyllum* Extract Ameliorates High-Fat Diet-Induced Obesity in C57BL/6N Mice by Upregulating SIRT1. *Nutrients.* 2019 Oct 15;11(10):2475.

182 Rao A, Clayton P, Briskey D. The effect of an orally-dosed Gynostemma pentaphyllum extract (ActivAMP) on body composition in overweight, adult men and women: A double-blind, randomised, placebo-controlled study. *J Hum Nutr Diet.* 2022 Jun;35(3):583-589.

183 Rahmani AH, et al. Implications of Green Tea and Its Constituents in the Prevention of Cancer via Modulation of Cell Signalling Pathway. *BioMed Res Int.* 2015 Apr 21;2015:925640.

184 Wiernsperger NF and Bailey CJ. The Antihypertensive Effect of Metformin. *Drugs.* 1999;58 Suppl 1:31-9; discussion 75-82.

185 Wang YW, et al. Metformin: a review of its potential indications. *Drug Des Devel Ther*. 2017;11:2421-2429.

186 Cork CK, et al. Real Talk: The Inter-play Between the mTOR, AMPK, and Hexos-amine Biosynthetic Pathways in Cell Signaling. *Fron Endocrinol (Lausanne)*. 2018;9:522.

187 Yang X, et al. Metformin, beyond an insulin sensitizer, targeting heart and pancreatic beta cells. *Biochim Biophys Acta Mol Basis Dis*. 2017 Sug;1863(8):1984-1990.

188 Schneider MB, et al. Prevention of pancreatic cancer induction in hamsters by metformin. *Gastroenterology*. 2001 Apr; 120(5):1263-70.

189 Libby G, et al. New users of metformin are at low risk of incident cancer: a cohort study among people with type 2 diabetes. *Diabetes Care*. 2009 Sep;32(9):1620-5.

190 National Institutes of Health (NIH): National Institute of Diabetes and Diges-tive and Kidney Diseases (NIDDKD): Overweight & Obesity Statistics. https://www.niddk.nih.gov/health-information/health-statistics/overweight-obesity

191 Stevanovic D, et al. Intracerebroventricular administration of metformin inhibits ghrelin-induced hypothalamic AMP-kinase signaling and food intake. *Neuroendocrinology*. 2012; 96: 24–31.

192 Adeyemo MA, et al. Effects of metformin on energy intake and satiety in obese children. *Diabetes Obes Metab*. 2014; 17: 363–370.

193 Chen C, et al. mTOR Regulation and Therapeutic Rejuvenation of Aging Hematopoietic Stem Cells. *Sci Signal*. 2009;2(98):ra75.

194 Chen C, et al. mTOR regulation and therapeutic rejuvenation of aging hema-topoietic stem cells. *Sci Signal*. 2009 Nov 24;2(98):ra75.

195 Urfer SR, et al. A randomized controlled trial to establish the effects of short-term rapamycin treatment in 24 middle-aged companion dogs. *Gero-Science*. 2017 Apr;39(2):117-127.

196 Dai DF, et al. Altered proteome turnover and remodeling by short-term caloric restriction or rapamycin rejuvenate the aging heart. *Aging Cell*. 2014 Jun;13(3):529-39.

197 Wallis LJ, et al. Demographic Change Across the Lifespan of Pet Dogs and Their Impact on Health Status. *Front Vet Sci*. 2018 Aug;23(5):200.

198 Urfer S, et al. A randomized controlled trial to establish effects of short-term rapamycin treatment in 24 middle-ages companion dogs. *GeroScience*. 2017 Apr 3;39:117-127.

199 Luo LL, Xu JJ, Fu YC. Rapamycin prolongs female reproductive lifespan. *Cell Cycle*. 2013;12(21):3353-3354.

INDEX